DEDICATION

Jesus - where would I be without your grace? This is a first fruit to you. I worship you with all my heart.

To my wonderful parents - words couldn't express how grateful and blessed I am to have you as our mum and dad. Everything I know about being a mum comes from your loving example.

To my dear Martin - the champion of my heart and my dreams. Thank you for giving me the confidence to write our daughter's story.

Teo's Timing

Cheryl Adamos Noutch

WAYMAKER BOOKS

Copyright © Cheryl Anne Adamos Noutch 2022

First published 2022 by Waymaker Books,

an Imprint of Sharpsword Studios, London

ISBN 978-1-9997985-9-8

The right of Cheryl Anne Adamos Noutch to be identified as the Author of the Work has been asserted by her in accordance with the Copyright, Designs and Patents Act 1988.

All rights reserved. No reproduction, copy, adaptation or transmission of this work may be made in any form without the written permission of the publisher.

Typeset in Centaur by Waymaker Books, London

Printed and bound by Ingram Spark

Cover Illustration by Cheryl Anne Adamos Noutch

CONTENTS

Foreword	7
Prologue	9
34 + 5 Days	11
High Dependency Unit	17
The Corridor	27
Cold Water, Narrow Table	29
Waymaker	33
Blurry Night	37
Day 0	41
Heel Prick Test	47
Bissy and Shirley	49
The Private Room - The Kindness of God	55
Little Clothes, Happy Visitors	61
A Father's Joy	67
DVT Socks and Delayed Discharge	71
DAY 6 - Scans, Weighing Scales and the NICU	77
Day 7 - The Turning Point	85
Day 8 - A Mother's Comfort	97

Day 9 - Battle Plan	103
The Minefield of Westfield	111
Day 10 - Rooming In	113
The First Night	119
Day 11 - Home at Last	121
The Fourth Trimester	125
The Goodness of God	127
The Time She Choked on Milk	131
Vulnerability Makes You Stronger	135
Don't Let Your Mind Wander into Lies	141
Dying to Self	145
"That C-Section Saved Our Lives, Cheryl!"	149
It Takes a Village	159
Forgiveness and Milestones	165

FOREWORD

For over 18 years, Cheryl and I have referred to each other as 'Dulin'. I'm not entirely sure the origins or backstory as to why we have this specific name but whenever I hear Cheryl refer to me as Afia, it seems slightly arbitrary and alien. We are Dulin to each other.

I think the simple way to define the word Dulin is by reading Proverbs 18:24b:

There is a friend who sticks closer than a brother.

Proverbs 18:24b is the essence of our relationship - the depth of our friendship - and I consider it an absolute honour to write this foreword and to prepare you to journey through this wonderful testament of the miraculous birth of Teodora Joy Christin Noutch.

It is common knowledge that a child is born every single minute of the day. Multiple births take place across the world and the human race continues to increase in number. Regardless of the statistics and how familiar we might become with birth stories, I believe that we should never take lightly that each child that transitions out of the womb is a miracle regardless of what route they take to enter the world. Birth is truly joyous.

In reading this book you will encounter the tremendous wonders of God and His faithfulness towards Cheryl and Martin on the birth of Teodora. You will hear the tenderness of a mother's heart, wisdom of a praying husband, strength birthed through vulnerability, the beautiful fragrance of praying parents, the purpose and importance of the Church family, the spiritual warfare over newborns and overall, the thanksgiving that can only come to faithful believers like Cheryl and Martin who trust in God in the face of uncertainty.

Not my will but yours be done.

This book is a reminder of what it truly means to lean on Jesus and die to self. We all need to be reminded that no matter what happens in life we can trust Him to care for us, our children and loved ones. We can trust God to provide for all our needs even if the circumstance is challenging and beyond our control. What a mighty God we serve!

I pray that you are blessed as you read this reflection on such a beautiful journey into motherhood, full of tender moments and spirit filled encounters. To God be the Glory for the things He has done.

Afia Yale, May 2021

PROLOGUE

Sixteen weeks and a day. The day I decided to write down the events and story of the birth of our darling Teo. Teodora Joy Christin Noutch. Our daughter. Our beloved gift from God - that's what her name means. As the days become more filled with her smiles, her growth and her milk-guzzling ways, her entry into the world becomes a romantic blur of precious moments. I don't want it to get lost in the haze of sleep deprivation and nappies. This is a testimony of birth: her miraculous delivery, my entry into motherhood and our growing family. God is incredibly good, merciful and loving, so I'm writing this story as an offering of thanksgiving for all He has done.

34 + 5 DAYS

34 weeks and 5 days was the day our daughter was born. I was 34 years and 5 months old when I became a mother. She was delivered by emergency caesarean-section because I had presented signs of high blood pressure and pre-eclampsia. Can I say I gave birth to her if she was cut from me? Yes - I can! *I should.*

"If we do not deliver this baby now, you could stroke. You could seizure - you could die. You and your baby are at risk."

At risk? Get her out. I turned to Martin, his face sombre and taking in the gravity of the words just spoken. Dr. James looked at us with calm and focus. I felt at peace.

"But she's only 34 weeks, it's too early. We were only discussing induction at 37 weeks this morning," Martin explained.

"Everything was fine this morning - my urine was clear. I have no headache - it's just a pain under my ribs - it hurts when I breathe."

As I said those words, I felt myself trying to justify why our baby girl should stay inside. *I knew she wasn't going to. And somehow I knew, I knew she would be early. But not this early.*

Doctor James replied quickly and with authority. "Even if all the evidence said that this morning, the evidence now is different. Your blood pressure has probably been worse than you thought all this time. We need to make a decision based on the evidence presented to us now. You have a trace of protein in your urine, your blood pressure is extremely high and you have a pain in your chest. These all point to pre-eclampsia. This baby is coming tonight."

I took Martin's hand and said, "We will see our baby girl tonight. It is well."

After that, I have no sense of time, only that Martin was there by my side. He rang my parents, his parents, our praying friends. We called the army to prayer. The only thought I had was - *she will be in my arms tonight.*

You're probably expecting my most spiritual outpouring and my deepest prayers to flow out in desperation - but honestly in that moment all I can say is - *I felt peace.* I knew that Jesus was with us. I know He had us in His hands. I knew He had already ordained the moments before, present and to come. We had no long prayer time or moment to compose ourselves.

We got on with it.

There was a chance that our daughter might need to be taken to the NICU (Neonatal Intensive Care Unit) because she would be premature. Her lungs and heart might not have formed properly yet. There could be all manner of complications. Martin was worried about having me and our daughter in two different places and how to attend to us both. All I could think was that none of that would happen. I had felt her move. I had felt the strength of her kicks. I knew she was strong. I knew her breathing would be fine.

Quite honestly, I felt as though I was in an episode of Holby City and that it was some kind of surreal dream. I sat there in a nippy hospital gown, surrounded by a Senior Consultant, two junior doctors, three midwives and my husband. Doris, the midwife, had promised to be with me the whole time. Doris who brought me DVT stockings and struggled to get them round my Filipino calves. It's amazing how quickly you latch onto some people as though you have always been friends. Doris felt to me like a big sister with a hearty laugh, a quick wit and a no-nonsense attitude. I felt she was fighting my corner.

An hour before, I was still at home contemplating whether or not to call triage. Earlier in the day we had met with our consultant who had organised a scan for the following morning because they were planning for me to be induced at

37 weeks. Martin was at work, tutoring and I went there because I thought I had indigestion. Four weeks previously, at week 30, I had been admitted with a headache and a slightly raised blood pressure. This time, as I was wheeled up to labour ward, I had to fight back fearful tears in the lift. "You will be alright, my dear," said Mary, the sister in charge. She wiped the tear from my face and brought me great assurance. Everything in my pregnancy till this point had been textbook and healthy.

My blood pressure was too high for even the machine to read. I needed to be injected with magnesium sulphate. I was told it would feel like a burning sensation as it hit my blood stream. The first doctor fitted a cannula. Doris was not pleased with his efforts. Though the situation seemed dangerous and life-threatening, I feel as though God helped me find the comedy. I have always felt that we - He and I - catch private jokes. My mind plays tricks with words and phrases and the tiniest interactions between people. The cut-eyes from Doris over the bloody mess the young doctor made had me stifling a giggle. My right wrist was sore, but I didn't pay any attention as I watched Dr. James take a large needle ready for my first dose.

"As soon as we have a window and your blood pressure goes down, we are delivering this baby."
Martin held my hand as the magnesium went in. It hit me instantly. I have never taken drugs, but I imagine this is what it would feel like. An alien substance fighting your blood. My

nerves were on fire. I began to sweat. It poured down my face. I was heating up. I am not a quiet person. I let everyone know it was burning. It was at this point that Martin thought it a good time to start singing, "Give me oil in my lamp, keep me burning."

The midwives in the room began to join in - I wasn't amused. My husband has a way with song. He finds a song for everything and does it with a loud voice. If you have heard him once, you won't forget his tone. The loudest English man in the room. The midwives enjoyed his entertainment. Dr. James watched my face intently to see how I was reacting. I thank God there were no mirrors in that space. Martin told me later I was turning purple, yellow, red and white.

Dr. James was calm. He paced the room and repeated again, *we just need a window*. I watched him: strangely, this was exciting. Not an ideal situation, no, but the doctor was excited. I suppose in this line of work, the scientist inside is intrigued with dilemma and scans the inner recesses of medical knowledge to find a quick solution. I've never had that kind of mind, but I imagine it to be a filing cabinet of alphabetised ailments, followed by firing arrows and mind maps of calculated risk and logic.

Dr James explained that he was born at 34 weeks and the other doctor in the room at 35. *So she might be a doctor one day.* I spoke aloud, trying to rouse a laugh from Martin. I could feel him thinking.

After that, Doris got me ready for theatre. I needed a catheter because of the c-section. Sorry to be graphic, but having a tube inserted into your nether regions is like trying to put a knife in a silk wrap case. It felt like a slicing pain. How I was ever going to push a baby out of there, I do not know! Doris tried twice, "Relax darling, relax, try to relax." The catheter was too painful. A catheter! She offered me gas and air. I love gas and air. It sent me into a laughing fit and I instantly thought about my brother. Wishing he was there to laugh with. No-one makes me laugh like my brother does.

Laughing uncontrollably - and at a high pitch - I was wheeled to the High Dependency Unit (HDU). My English gent was embarrassed by my show! You have to find the funny moments in these situations. Therein lies humanity. The doctors asked what had happened to me. Doris - dead pan and looking like she'd had enough of me at this point -said, "I gave her gas and air."

"For what?" said the most bemused doctor.

"A catheter."

I didn't see the doctor's face, but I imagine he thought I was a lightweight.

HIGH DEPENDENCY UNIT

I sobered up pretty quickly in the HDU. The mood was serious and dark. It was evening. I had left behind the private room of the labour ward and its comforts. The midwives on this ward were busy and serious and didn't smile. They moved in and out of bays quickly and quietly, holding precious information for recording into documents moments later.

For a moment, Martin and I could turn to each other and pray. We called on God and encouraged our hearts in the Word. The sonic aid was strapped to my pregnant belly, picking up baby girl's heartbeat. The gushing movements of her swishing brought me comfort and hope. I knew she was strong. I knew I was fine. After 34 weeks, I had gotten to know this unknown being. I'd lie awake at night counting her kicks obsessively and I'd rub my belly talking to her when I snuck to the kitchen for snacks. Now, I was told she was showing signs of distress. I didn't believe it. I knew she was strong. I rubbed her still and spoke words of life over her. Psalms flooded my mind.

You spend all this time preparing. Pregnancy is a joyful and unstable time in a woman's body. They say the third trimester the hardest. That week I had just begun packing my hospital bag. I have no shame in telling you that all I had anticipated was a night's observation in the hospital, so all I'd packed was a pair of knickers and my Bible. I was so grateful I hadn't left the house without His Word.

Martin took my hand. I cannot remember his words. I just know he was covering me in prayer. My parents had arrived but were not allowed into the HDU. How I longed to see them. Knowing they were close was enough. I knew my mum would be worried and daddy would be reassuring her. We had Psalm 139 open. We read over our baby. We spoke these scriptures over her:

> *For you formed my inward parts;*
> *You covered me in my mother's womb.*
> *I will praise You, for I am fearfully and wonderfully made;*
> *Marvellous are Your works,*
> *And that my soul knows very well.*
> *My frame was not hidden from You,*

When I was made in secret,
And skilfully wrought in the lowest parts of the earth.
Your eyes saw my substance, being yet unformed.
And in Your book they all were written,
The days fashioned for me,
When as yet there were none of them.

How precious are your thoughts to me, O God!
How great is the sum of them!
If I should count them, they would be more in number than the sand;
When I awake, I am still with You."

Psalm 139: 13-18

And somewhere, His strength filled us. All Martin and I could focus on in those moments was praying for each other, for our baby and for the nurses and doctors who would be with us. We made a promise to each other in that darkened HDU that we would bless every midwife, doctor and nurse that we came into contact with. We recognised that in our deepest moment of need, God was calling us to serve and worship Him through it. We were to find the praise in the hard place. We didn't know exactly what we were promising God just before surgery, but we knew He would make good on that promise.

Before the signing of official documents and explanation of possible complications and procedures, our first testing of that promise came when one of the midwives overheard us praying. She asked us for prayer. In that moment, she brought her deepest desire before me and Martin and asked us to pray. So we did - we prayed for her. Doris told her off. "This is not a time to pray." *Every single moment is a time of prayer.*

We prayed a blessing over her future and the desires of her heart - I know it was a God appointment.

She scuttled off into the night reprimanded by my dear Doris. Doris was my guardian, not allowing anyone to stress me or come near. Praise God for Doris.

Martin and I flipped through Psalm 127, 91, 135, 121 - words of comfort, of strength, of deliverance. A week before, I had not slept much. God had prepared my heart in scriptures. Scriptures I had post-it-noted above my side of the bed. Words that now flowed from my lips and girded my heart.

I will deliver you.

Psalm 91: 15

And the Lord stood by me and strengthened me.
2 Timothy 4:17

When my heart is overwhelmed, lead me to the rock that is higher than I.

Psalm 61: 2

When you feel the crushing of the world's air around you - it is then you realise what fragrance is released from within you. I don't say this to boast in my own merit but to declare that God had promised He would deliver us. In every sense of the word.

Dr. Duncan - a sweet Ghanaian man, softly spoken and light-hearted, came to explain spinal anaesthesia. Oddly enough he reminded me of daddy. My daddy is an anaesthetist. Again I felt God's favour somehow. I felt that the Lord was bringing us comfort. In His infinite wisdom, He had orchestrated and handpicked the exact team and the correct group of people to be with us. Doris the guardian, Dr. James the strategist and now Dr. Duncan - someone I could trust with a needle in my spine.

He explained the numbing of my nerves and inserting of a needle like instructions for fixing a bell on a child's bike.

A simple procedure. Nothing to worry over. Some women shake, some women vomit, some do not. It is all normal. You won't feel your legs for up to 48 hours. You will be paralysed from the ribs down. But don't worry: it's normal.

I appreciated his manner. He read me the one-in-10-million chance of this and 1-in-100-million chance of that. Yes he put me at ease - but, wow, did I not want to let myself dwell on the what-ifs.

You can have as much faith, as much Word and as much Jesus in your life, but deep down we are still human, and fear and worry is a very real enemy. This is the other side of the coin, if we choose to flip it. A hospital is a flip-coin place, where fear and faith battle in the atmosphere; hope and disappointment both loom. It takes more than positive words and kind intentions to turn a heart towards joy in a place like that. It takes Jesus.

Dr Amy (one of the other doctors who had been attending us earlier) returned just as Martin and I were reading through more scripture and holding hands. We stopped. She told us to continue. She waited till we finished before talking to us.

How respectful. She was calm and logical and very professional. She filled me with confidence. I could read her face and she was reading mine.

She explained that my baby's heart rate was slowing down and showing signs of distress. *I didn't believe her words.* I would need a steroid injection as a precaution to support babies lungs in case her breathing was weak. I accepted every help I was offered: I wanted to give her the best. Dr. Amy disappeared and a nurse returned with the injection.

"Sharp scratch."

More pain. I don't know what was worse: the burning of the magnesium sulphate injection or the steroid jab that felt like a mighty blow to my outer thigh and painful suction in my muscles. It felt as though a bruise had formed in seconds. The flow of the steroid jab brought a painful shiver up my leg. It wasn't till a few days later I noticed the black and blue bruising.

Dr. Amy came back a few moments later, it wouldn't be long now before I had the caesarean. They were preparing the theatre for me. She pre-empted every question I had before I asked it. Martin and I were still hoping we could somehow stall this moment and keep baby girl inside longer. She very carefully and tactfully said, "This is the safest option for your baby now."

I wanted to know about my birthing plan - the plan you write as though you could really control how you could have your baby. I, like many other women, had dreamed of a water birth, with dimmed lights, music and hands-off treatment from midwives. It would just be me and Martin and Jesus. How stark in contrast this moment was. Doctor Amy explained that Martin wouldn't be able to cut the cord, that I wouldn't be able to see the procedure. I would be veiled behind a cloth and my baby might be able to come to the ward with me depending on her state when she was delivered. At that point, the only thing I wanted was to feel God's presence. To feel His steadying hand, His assurance that everything would be well.

Could I play music?

"Of course, if you have something to play it on," was Doctor Amy's reply.

The only thing that was true to the birth plan was the playing of worship music. This - like only coming out of the house with a pair of knickers and a bible - was the only thing on His agenda, to worship. We were leaning and trusting in Him through all of this.

What followed was the formality of paperwork. Dr. Amy brought the papers to explain the procedure and all that could happen. It's a strange feeling giving your consent to a procedure you only understand in part, placing your trust in someone to surgically deliver your baby, all the while not knowing if it will be straight forward. Martin reminded me - my trust is secure in the Lord and that's where we were to look.

Dr Amy, how many c-sections have you successfully performed?

"Around a thousand," she replied, turning her back to me as she walked out of the cubicle. I breathed a sigh of relief. She was steady, I liked her calm.

Martin went to tell mum and dad that I was being prepared for theatre. Doris came back to prepare the bed for transport. I desperately wanted to see my parents.

Can I see them? Doris had my back. Doctor Duncan appeared too. Martin went to change into scrubs. He came back having seen mum and dad. They had prayed together and mum had said, "Don't worry, Holy Spirit is with you."

Oh to hear the words of a praying mum. They clad your heart with the strongest rock. Strength filled me afresh. I believe she felt the same knowledge of her daughter that I felt for the baby girl growing in my womb. *She is strong and full of life.*

THE CORRIDOR

Doris and Doctor Duncan and another midwife wheeled me out of the HDU and the Labour Ward reception. I would later grow accustomed to the layout and through doors linking the HDU to the NICU. Doris had squared it with security for my parents to see me before theatre. I sat in the bed at the mercy of the doctors and nurses, Martin by my side. I was wheeled round the corner and there they stood. My mum and dad.

Doctor Duncan - my dad and mum. This is my dad. He is an anaesthetist like you.

I watched their exchange - like soldiers of the field sharing a knowing glance. My daddy locked eyes with him and said, "You look after my daughter, give her the best." They shook hands.

"Yes, sir."

They came to me. Daddy took my hand and kissed me. Mummy my other hand. I knew that if I cried, she would too. I smiled instead and told her it would be ok. She told me she was praying. All I felt was love. Here they were - my parents. My rocks. My champions. And there we were, Martin and I, on the verge of also being handed the mystery of loving a child. It was more than words could express.

It was as though the bed didn't pause between the HDU and theatre. Doris had taken off her weave. *Is that a surgery cap?*

She laughed, "No! It's too hot, I had to take off my hair."

COLD WATER, NARROW TABLE

Ever had surgery? In 34 years of life, never had I ever needed to see the doctor for anything more than a stubborn sore throat from terms of teaching, a dodgy right ankle and skin allergies. I hadn't seen any doctors in my pregnancy until week 30. Pregnancy is surprisingly doctor-less if you are 'low risk'. And here I was, about to be surrounded by more doctors than I had ever met in my whole lifetime.

A cherry-cheeked young doctor came to introduce himself.

"Hello, I am the baby doctor. I will be here checking your baby after she comes out."

"Nice to meet you, baby doctor, what is your name?"

"Doctor Angus."

God bless Doctor Angus.

I needed to be transferred from hospital bed to the operating table. The table was thin. Thinner than me.

How will I fit on that table for the surgery?

"Will you be with me in the surgery Doris?"

"I won't leave you darling. I will be with you all the way."

She stood in front of me, my hands on her shoulders. Her hands pressed the band of the sonic aid - we were still monitoring the baby's heartbeat. All the while, her heart rate in the background swishing and sloshing away. My ear was always on it. My hands protectively on my belly - my girl. Doctor Duncan and two other anaesthetists were preparing frantically behind me. I was sat on the thin table, my legs dangling over the edge and being asked to bend forward to elongate my spine.

Prickly, cold sprays.

"Can you feel the spray?"

"Why do you have to use cold water? Why can't you use warm water?"

I understand the logic of being sprayed to check your feeling - but who wants to be cold?

Doris held me in place. Doctor Duncan showed me the needle. I never want to see a needle like that again. It looked as long as a 30cm ruler. I'll never look at a ruler length without thinking of that needle again. It probably wasn't that long - I'm no good at estimating length.

Then, just like that, I couldn't feel my legs. I could see them and I tried to tell them to move. But they would not obey. It intrigued me. I was sprayed again - I felt nothing. Nothing!

I was swung round and laid down on the table. The thin table had swung sides. My arms were strapped out like Jesus on the cross. How surreal. There I was, lying down in cross position, surrendered to them. Trusting that God would use them to save me and my child. My blood pressure, heart rate and the sonic aid were running through the different machines. *Where was Martin?*

More nurses came in, midwives and, I think, a baby doctor team. *Where were the doctors? Where was Martin?*

Doctor Duncan wasn't happy, I had been waiting on the table for five minutes, but no doctors were appearing to operate on me. I looked up at the operating lights and read the markings on them. The lights were called 'Martin' lights. Again I asked where my husband was. Someone went to find him. At this point, I counted at least 15 people in the room. A blue curtain was put in front of my face. It was incredibly claustrophobic.

The doors swung open - there he was - my Martin. He walked over to me and sat next to me. I love my husband, when he walks into the room something in me settles, I feel safe knowing he is there in every situation. I beckoned for his hand. He had my phone. I told him I wanted the worship music on. The doctors arrived. I looked to my right - there was Doris now with a surgical cap on and Doctor Duncan sat behind my head. I had begun to shake - I was cold. I was not comfortable. I wanted to be sick. The blue cloth was in my face. I felt I couldn't breathe. The whole evening, I had felt a pain under my ribs like I had tied a belt on too tight. Earlier, Doctor James had said the pain was a sign my liver was breaking down. Right now, I couldn't feel it. In fact, because of the anaesthesia, I couldn't feel the end of my breath in my lungs. I kept imagining that the bottom of my lungs had fallen off like an aeroplane blown in half in the middle of a flight. I wanted to puke.

All I knew was that Doctor Amy and Doctor James were there. I suppose the other people in the room were student doctors, midwives and nurses. The baby team were there ready and waiting. I looked to my right and watched the two midwives watching the doctors. I was shaking the whole time. I couldn't control it. Doctor Duncan was talking to me and holding my head, Martin my hand. They hadn't even started yet and I was unable to control the shakes. I turned to Martin.

Please play the playlist. The list we had prepared for the birth.

"Do you want me to play all of it?" Martin asked.

We only have time for one - Way Maker.

WAYMAKER

Ladies. Mothers to be. Women in waiting. Pray for a man who loves God. Pray for a man who will fight for His wife when she has no words to admit she needs him. I know I joked about having a husband whose voice is the loudest in the room, and if you hear his tone you will never forget it.

I never felt so safe and assured as I did then. Hearing Martin's voice above the beeps and monitors. His loud, comforting sound sung the first two lines.

As he sang, I heard a voice above my head start joining in, like warm water pouring over my head. It was Doctor Duncan. Then another voice from my right side.

It was Doris - and another midwife, whose name I would later find was Sherell. I wish I could tell you I was singing along at the top of my lungs being extremely brave and focusing on Jesus. But I was not - I was shaking, I was trying to breath. My worship to Him was my breath. Doctor Duncan was trying to calm me down. I just wanted to vomit. Martin held my hand, tried to keep the blue cloth from my face as he kept singing.

By the chorus, more voices had joined in. I don't know who and I won't remember their faces. But I felt Him. I felt God there. There He was, through these wonderful people. There He was in the middle of an operating room in Newham General Hospital. There He was holding my hand through my husband. There He was in the atmosphere as the people sang and lifted up His name. This was the perfect atmosphere for our girl to be born. I looked up at the Martin light beaming above me and the grey ceiling tiles. Thank you Jesus.

Martin's head shot up. I looked at him.

"Did you hear that? That was a cry."

The room was singing and humming.

Turn the music off.

Cries. Loud, strong, lungs-full-of-air cries. My baby. My girl. I heard her before I saw her. I heard her voice.

I had managed to stop shaking by this point, I had been pumped with some kind of anti-sickness medication three times during what seemed like ten minutes. Doctor Duncan explained I was now being sewn up. It's hard to explain, that I felt her being pulled from me, but I did not feel pain. I felt my insides being pushed and moved, squished and tugged - but no pain. A strange sensation. It was secondary to the shaking and shuddering.

I watched Martin's face. I watched him watching the baby

team.

What is happening?

"They're checking her."

Go to her.

Martin went over to the baby doctor. He took a photo and brought the photograph to me. I cried. Relief. She was here. Pink and angry looking. And so she should be. Plucked from a safe place. Pulled before her due date. But I was so glad. I just wanted to hold her. Our precious girl.

Go and hold her. She needs to hear your voice.

Martin went over. He asked to hold her and Doctor Angus let him. Martin spoke to her, assured her. It was right. She heard my voice all those weeks, every day and every night. The first voice she heard on the outside was her father's voice. Her first hug was her father's hug. The revelation of the Father heart of God will stay with me forever as I think of this. What manner of child is this? That she would be born to the sound of worship and that God would choose Martin's to be the first hold and hug she felt. That somehow, she will grow to know something so special about the Father's love through this moment.

"Can my wife hold her?"

Doctor Angus was still looking at her vital signs. Her skin tone, the colour of her cheeks. He was tracking her breathing, her heart rate - any signs of distress. Doctor Angus brought her to me. Wrapped in a towel. I was still on the operating table. Martin was next to me once more. He brought her close to my face.

Hello baby girl. I love you. Well done baby girl. Mummy loves you.

I kissed her face. She turned her head to my voice. I cried a whole lot more. Overjoyed.

Doctor Angus gave the ok for our baby girl to come to the HDU with me. All 1.9kgs of her. Martin had her in his arms as I was placed back into the hospital bed. Doris took her from Martin and placed her into my arms. My girl in my arms. I will never forget that moment. From feeling sick and not seeing beyond the blue veil, to cradling this precious baby in my arms. She felt so light, so tiny. Her little eyes were closed and her pink cheeks looked so fresh.

All that talk about her lungs not being strong - there she was in my arms content. Oh how she proved them wrong. Miraculous. My God truly - a WAYMAKER!

BLURRY NIGHT

I was wheeled back to the HDU to the same bay, the same blue curtains, the same feeling of no air in the room. I had no idea what time it was. I hadn't eaten since lunch time. I was thirsty. My mouth was dry. There was a baby girl in my arms. She was asleep. She was mine. So beautiful. I had brought nothing for her. No clothes, no nappies. Nothing to show for the last 4 weeks of washing, ironing and nesting. Nothing to prove I had done the preparing. She was wrapped in towels.

In my mind it was still 9pm - the time I arrived at the hospital. Time had seemed to stand still, go slow and pass quickly all the same. Our darling girl was delivered at 1:03am. As I was wheeled back to the HDU, I asked Doris if I could see my parents. She wouldn't budge, "You need to rest now."

I looked down at this sweet bundle of joy, eyes closed and still. All I could do was stare. Martin was still in scrubs and was walking alongside me. We got settled in the HDU and Martin started to arrange things close around me. Water, phone, phone charger, bible, blanket. I started to feel drowsy. I wasn't allowed to drink or eat anything for another 12 hours. I was expecting to spend the first night as a family in this blue, windowless cocooned bay - however one midwife explained that partners were not allowed to stay and that visiting hours stopped at 9pm. My heart sank - I wanted him with me and our baby.

He dutifully obeyed. We discussed what he would bring for the morning - I had only just started packing my hospital bag that week. I am quite proud to say, in my pregnancy nesting, I'd sectioned the baby drawers into size order from left to right and what he needed would be the first row of clothes for her in the left hand side of the drawer (I'd like to say it is still like this but that would be a lie).

It was uncomfortable sitting in the bed, I was beginning to regain feeling in the lower half of my body - which felt like a slow release from pins and needles from the waist down. It didn't matter - our daughter was alive and in my arms. Martin was almost ready to go, his green jacket and flat cap set. He sat on the bed and drew me and baby girl close. The lights were dimmed on the ward.

"I don't want us to wait too long to name her. What shall we name her?"

We had spent the pregnancy not really agreeing on names. We both knew it needed a worshipful meaning. I had even bought *The Complete Book of Baby Names* a few weeks earlier and we had spent an evening laughing through the many lists. By this point we had shortlisted around six names and had decided we would wait to meet her before we penned her full name.

It is a sacred moment, naming your child. People's opinions and values over names tell you much about their tolerance and experience for people. We held this short list close to our hearts and shared it with no-one. We didn't want her name gunned down before she had even had a chance to use it. Nor did we want anyone else calling her other names in the meantime.

We looked down at her and one name came into my heart. This sweet being, a gift from God Himself, bringing us such joy out of such a circumstance. Teodora.

And Martin smiled and agreed. Just a few days prior, we had spent the afternoon in the garden at my mum and dads or Little Philippines as Martin and I call it. The kind of garden that made me feel I was back home, where you sit under the shade with dad playing Spanish guitar. I was ordered to sit on a chair and put my feet up. I had desperately wanted to garden and plant flowers. My dad wouldn't allow it and neither would Martin or mummy. So I sat on a chair, balancing a plate of watermelon on my belly, eating happily and enjoying being so round that I was ordered to rest. *This is the best bit about pregnancy. Not being allowed to lift a finger.*

Martin and daddy had been burning old bits of wood. We'd

sat around the fire till it got too cold even with our cardigans and coats. Whilst mummy and I were inside, Daddy and Martin had discussed names. Dads suggestion was Christin - "It's like Martin and Cheryl mixed together and also Christ-in you, Christ-in Noutch." We loved Daddy's thoughtfulness and had decided that night it would be one of her names.

There she was Teodora Joy Christin Noutch - her daddy overjoyed to be able to call her by name the first time we prayed together as a family of three. Jesus was there in the midst of us, holding hands and holding each other. We dedicated her life to Him that night and prayed thanks for giving us this beloved gift.

DAY 0

Martin decided he would walk from Newham General all the way home. If you know my husband, you know he loves to walk. He walks when he needs to chew on thoughts, projects and book ideas. He walks to feel connected to Jesus. He walks when he needs to feel alive and refreshed again. He walks to worship. That night - I knew is walk would be a victorious giving of thanks walk. I waited for his text to let me know he was home.

In the midst of all that went on, we had an army of saints - family and friends praying for us. Prayer, I believe that petitioned the Heavens and called down provision for strength, hope, peace, mercy and divine health. Prayers that sent angels to our aid and Jesus Himself to the operating room. Prayers that brought the right doctors and nurses to our side. Prayers that covered me, Martin and Teodora as a family beginning our journey as a three. It is only now, weeks on that I recognise the magnitude of what we faced. It could have been a very different story. I faced my own mortality and Martin had to pray a prayer that a husband and soon-to-be father should never have to pray. What was asked of us that night, was to totally surrender to God our lives as we knew it and to be willing to worship through the uncertainty. I had given Martin the task of letting everyone know we were alright. I am so thankful to the church. I know many people have many stories of how they were hurt by the church - but this is not our experience. Our church family rallied, pressed in and prayed for our daughter like she was their own. This speaks to me of His kindness. Praise God.

Between sending Martin home and settling down for the night, the midwives were switching shifts. One nurse came to introduce herself - her name was Bissy. Softly spoken and sweet natured she picked up Teodora like she was the most precious baby in the world. She introduced herself and noticed that Teo had no clothes. I explained that Martin would bring some in the morning because I didn't know I was having my baby that night.

"Don't worry mummy, it's ok. We will wrap her up warm," her melodious Caribbean accent calmed my anxiety.

She wrapped Teo in a towel, then a hospital blanket and placed her delicately on her side in the cot. Moments later a nurse from the NICU came to see us. She had brought a knitted white hat and a tiny baby sleep suit. Praise God - my baby is getting dressed. Teo did not like the cold. She let us know about it. I was proud to hear her cry. It filled me with so much hope. Those lungs were expressing praise to God. She was crying out on the breathe He had given her.

It was the smallest hat I had ever seen and it was still too big for her 4 pound 3 ounce frame. I folded it over to make it sit so that it didn't cover her eyes. She seemed to like being warm on her head. The tiny baby suit was loose and hanging off her. Her little arms were folding inside the sleeves. She wanted to curl up. Every instinct in me wanted to wrap her up and keep her close to my bosom. Just hours before, she was still inside me, enjoying the warmth and safety of my womb. I wrapped the hospital blanket around her tiny frame and watched her nestle and stir in my arms. Her smell was delicious. It melted my heart. The smell of my baby. I suppose that is the smell of vernix. I had hoped they wouldn't wipe all of it away but I later learned that because my liver and kidneys were breaking down, there was a high chance of infection in the placenta. They had to wipe Teo clear for risk of infection.

That night, my little Teo needed me. Born at 34 weeks and 5 days, I didn't know if I even had milk for her. I knew I was sore and that my shape had changed. Much reading told me that some women experience their milk coming in the weeks before their babies are born. I was not one of those women. Bissy, the midwife, encouraged me to try. Teodora was beginning to root. To look for milk. Her cry was music to my ears. This little being, whose soft yelps brought tears to my eyes. I didn't care for the cut below my belly button, or the tingling sensation in the nerves of my legs - all I could think of was wanting to give my daughter what she needed.

Bissy helped me hold Teodora into position and she latched for the first time. Ouch.

I did not care about the soreness. All I knew was that my daughter was trying to feed. I had no understanding of how it should feel or even if she was taking anything from me. That night, I was breast-feeding for the first time. My girl was hungry and I was doing the most natural thing a mother could do. Bissy left me to it.

No sooner had Bissy left than Teo came off. I tried the other side - but she just fell asleep. I wondered if she'd had anything. I felt the questions arise.

Did she get anything? Is she full already? What if there is no milk in there? Was my milk enough?

That night, Bissy, Barbra and Sherelle attended to me multiple times. I was exhausted. Bissy came back to check on my progress. "Did she drink?"

I think so. Can we give her some formula? I am not sure if I have any milk?

Bissy went off to find some. I had read that they could live off the amniotic fluid for another 10 hours after being born, but being the rice-loving Filipino I am, I wanted to make sure my daughter was full. I was exhausted. I remember falling in and out of sleep that night. Teodora slept mostly in my arms.

Absolute bliss.

HEEL PRICK TESTS

Doctor Angus (who I had called Agnes several times in the operating theatre) appeared to check on Teodora. Her poor little left foot, pricked for blood samples to check her blood sugar levels and signs of infection. He listened to her heart and observed her skin. He made her suck on his gloved finger and checked for tongue tie. He was pleased with her progress. Her blood sugars were at the right level. He explained she needed to clear for signs of infection in the next 2 tests. I liked him - he attended to Teodora like a patient, telling her what he was doing and speaking to her like she understood what was happening. He treated her like she understood him. And I could tell she didn't mind him. He explained that she would need a cannula so that they could take samples and give medicine if they needed to. Teodora showed her utter disagreement with the needle and fought and cried. "She is a strong one!" Doctor Angus exclaimed.

It was a miracle that she was with me in the HDU at all that night. Most babies born with low-birth weight and that early are transported to the NICU (Newborn Intensive Care Unit).

The truth is, you really don't know the strength of a baby's heart and lungs till they are born into the world. We later found out that Teodora was in shock when she was delivered from me. She wasn't breathing straight away. She went from 0% blood oxygen saturation to 100% in the first 2 minutes and after that continued to show signs of progress. I thank God I didn't know these things straight away. Again, the Lord knew what we could handle and when we could handle them. Martin's prayer had been answered. She was not separated from us.

I drifted in and out of sleep.

Another doctor appeared in between the midwives trying to help me to feed. He didn't rub Teo's foot like Dr. Angus did or speak to her like a patient - she cried and seemed so angry. A fierce protective instinct rose from the inside of me. I told the doctor to leave her alone and come back after she'd had some sleep. I think he saw my face and reasoned it was better to listen to me as mama. Martin says I have a bad cop complex when it comes to talking to people. He assumes good cop naturally. I secretly hoped that Dr. Angus would come back to do the other tests.

That first night moved quickly, my blood pressure was monitored as I drifted in and out of sleep, in between feeds and heel prick tests. I watched the light change on the ceiling and bounce off the royal blue bay curtains. I couldn't wait to see Martin again. Now all I wanted was to go home.

BISSY AND SHIRLEY

This story isn't complete without writing about the midwives we met, the way they loved us and cared for us. They became the friendliest faces to me throughout this whole journey. They understood the journey we were on without me having to explain, they were on our side and they kept the place lively!

That first morning when the lights went on, I looked over at the baby cot next to me. I was groggy. I must have slept for some of it, I vaguely remember Bissy feeding Teodora some formula. Baby girl was sleeping peacefully on her side, her cheeks still pink and warm. My girl. My baby. Bissy was my Nightingale, so quiet and peaceful. A very sweet woman - my heart was glad to have her around on the first night. Her presence greatly encouraged me that first night.

I could hear the midwives handing over and talking in the front of the HDU first thing in the morning. Beeps and machines were firing up and down the room, the HDU was a noisy place. A place I would grow well acquainted with. My phone was going off with congratulations and texts were coming in left right and centre. I was glad that the signal in the room was weak, I couldn't handle phone calls just yet. Martin had sent a photo of me and Teo out to all our family and friends and was handling the communication which was all fine for me. My brother was in the Philippines and he thought I was joking. He wasn't expecting his niece to be an early bird. Those first messages from people were so beautiful.

I was so thirsty, I was thankful when I saw the lady coming round to take orders for breakfast. The whole night, whilst Teo was having checks, midwives were coming in to monitor my blood pressure. My hope was that it would come right down and that I was out of danger. Despite the soreness where my scar was, I was feeling good.

In the distance, I heard a friendly voice, a chipper good morning and introduction at the front. My Martin had come bringing my hospital bag, some food and supplies for our girl. My heart leapt to hear him. He came around the corner and greeted us - his girls. We had our download (our "What's been happening?" catch up) - even though we had only seen each other a few hours before.

A little Asian lady popped her head around the curtain to introduce herself for the day - her name was Shirley. We got acquainted and Martin got talking with her. She told me that I would have to start moving and walking! Walking - after seven layers of skin, tissue, muscle and nerves had been cut through. She explained that I was to put my weight on my arms to at least sit up, so that my legs could start to move again. I later learned that after a c-section it's important to get mobile, it lowers the risk of blood clots in the leg. I managed to sit at the end of the bed. She tried to get me to get up and sit on the chair next to the bed. I couldn't manage that then. She said not to worry and that we would try again later.

By this time breakfast was on its way, that two pieces of toast with jam and hot cup of tea felt like a Michelin restaurant English breakfast with all the trimmings. That tea filled me with a fresh strength. That first day was chilled - Martin and I took turns to sing to and carry Teo. I carried on feeding and getting to know how to feed her. We took photos of her and just stared at her. Whether you have faith or not - babies are miraculous. All that power and might displayed in a weak, tender babe completely dependent on your help and love.

Shirley was brilliant - she kept checking in on us. We found out she was a Christian and she blessed our baby. She commented on how strong Teodora was even though she was so tiny. When we changed her - she gave a loud cry, she kicked those little legs and let us know she didn't like being disturbed from her sleep. I know the NHS has a policy of not talking about religion, so I must point out here, at no point did any of the midwives or doctors tell us about their faith, we were the nosy ones. So I don't think they broke any rules in answering our questions. It was comforting to us to know we were surrounded by brothers and sisters in Christ.

We had many of the team from the night before come and see us. Doctor Angus came back with results and told us that Teodora had cleared her heel prick tests, Doctor Duncan the anaesthetist came to see us first thing and I prayed for him. I was so grateful for his care and experienced hand in looking after me. At every opportunity we could say thank you - we did.

It was the doctors we were waiting on. Doctor Amy, Doctor James and Doctor Matt came in the midmorning to check on us. They were very happy with how everything went and Doctor James said it was the right call. I had noticed a scratch on Teo's head and she explained that Teo needed forceps to be delivered and that she had seemed shocked when she came out. I looked down at my little darling and thanked the Lord again for His hand of deliverance. He had promised that He would deliver her and He did.

I asked when I could go home - my heart sank when Doctor James explained that it could be 3 or 4 days as my blood pressure was in a state of fluctuation because of the c-section and medication I was now on. It was our prayer point from then on in. I needed to relax and just let the medication take its course.

That first day - Day 0 - was precious. What I remember most was holding Teodora in my arms and just being overwhelmed with love. A love I didn't know I could express or feel for any other human being. I know people talk about this and you read about it. But suddenly my mum's words became real, "One day you will have children Cheryl and you know will know..." Words that she had spoken to me growing up when I was disobedient but now words I clung to, in awe of my mother's love.

It's a love that made me think about the scripture - "If you being evil know how to give good gifts to your children, how much more your Father in heaven." Oh I wept. The goodness of God to let me experience an ounce of the love he feels for His children whilst I held this little girl in my arms. I was proud of her without her even achieving a thing, I was fiercely protective even though no-one had laid a finger of harm on her, I was ready to do anything to keep her safe and happy even if she had no understanding of me being mama. That must be how it feels to be called a child of God and to be loved by Him.

THE PRIVATE ROOM - THE KINDNESS OF GOD

The 2nd day in the HDU was much like the first, noisy, eventful. You're surrounded by these royal blue curtains separating you from other new parents and their babies and you speak in hushed tones so as not to make your private thoughts known to the whole room with 5 bays, 5 mothers & 5 baby cots. There was every type of mother in there. The one whose blood pressure was too low, the one who had pre-eclampsia, the one with the dangerous positioning of the placenta, the one whose baby was in the NICU and then there was me, the one with high blood pressure and the baby with low birth weight.

Martin and I love people watching. In this case, it was people listening. You try to not listen in when the doctors do their rounds but you soon grow bored staring at blue curtains. We winced hearing husbands argue with the midwives because they couldn't stay with their wives, we laughed when we heard Sherell (the midwife who was in the operating theatre with us) reprimand a dad for calling her rude, "How am I being rude when I am telling the rules of the visiting hours?" But mostly, we cuddled up together the three of us. The three of us. How sweet to now be a three.

That second morning in the HDU I was feeling stronger. Bissy had once again supported me through the night. Quite a few midwives had come to check on me, it felt a bit like Piccadilly Circus with hearing tests, heel prick tests, blood pressure checks and general questions like, "How many wet nappies mum?" and "Is she feeding from you?" I was glad to see the light change in the room from night to dawn and then the day. I longed to be outside.

The feisty Caribbean midwife, Sherelle, came to greet me and tell me that today I would be walking and taking a shower. I looked at her in disbelief! Did she not know I had had an emergency c-section and that I was attached still to the catheter that Doris so carefully fitted? Judging by how she had dealt with angry dad - I realised I would not be able to argue with her. She seemed firm whilst still being caring. She came over to me, told me to sit up and walk to the chair.

"You can do it mum, I was there in the operating room. You were the one we sang Waymaker over the baby."

In that moment, I looked over at her with such gratitude. We gave each other a knowing look. She came over to inspect Teodora and spoke to her. She commented on how strong she was when she heard her cry. Everyone seemed to say this about her.

I couldn't help but think of how the Lord handpicked each person to help us in this time. Martin had arrived to find Sherelle supporting me to sit in the chair and bring Teodora over to me for a cuddle. He was glad to see me sitting up. I don't remember how but Sherelle left us singing "To God be the glory great things He has done." A hymn we heard belted out throughout the day. It was the hymn Martin sang when Teodora was placed in his arms in the delivery room.

That day, we met Maria, the Filipino midwife who had lost her voice. Once again, the Lord showed his kindness through his sense of humour - sending me a fellow countryman, an ate (big sister). Sherelle removed the catheter and handed me over to Maria. Often when I meet other Filipinos, they don't know that I am Filipino. Martin gave me away by saying, "Good morning Ate!" That whole day, he teased her for not having a speaking voice and she kept playfully poking him and calling him, "Makulet" the closest translation for that is cheeky troublemaker.

It was time for my first shower - Sherelle had said, "You will feel so much better afterwards, I promise you." Maria explained I needed to be careful with my scar and to not put soap on it. This would be the first time I would see myself in the mirror since Wednesday. It was now Friday morning. Bissy, who had been with me for two nights, graciously walked me to the bathroom. A mere 20 steps. 20 steps that felt like 20 miles. Martin looked after Teo whilst I went to shower.

I did everything so slowly. I was so glad for the seat in the shower. I thought that I would feel shock seeing my body for the first time. I have always had hang-ups about my figure, I am sure everyone does. But as I looked and studied my tummy, where my baby girl once lived and how my swollen face and hands had subsided - I was thankful. For the first time in my life, I felt such pride in my body. I had carried a baby for 34 weeks and 5 days. My body had housed the miraculous. I felt strong. I am not ashamed I cried happy tears in the shower. Sherelle was right - I felt so much better afterwards.

We were visited by Doctor James again - he explained that I needed to try and relax. My blood pressure had come down well but was spiking every now and again - so they had to monitor me to find the right combination of medication to keep it steady. He said that it was normal for the body to do this because it is realising that there was no more baby inside the womb, my body was readjusting. He was confident that I would be able to go home in a couple of days.

Shortly afterwards our Ate Maria came to tell us that they would be moving me downstairs to Larch Ward to a private room. Once again we felt the Lord's kindness. We had done the walk round before Teo was born with lots of expectant parents and seen the delivery suite, the rooms with pools, the wards with bays and the private rooms. Private rooms that you had to pay £80 a night for. We wouldn't have to pay because I was coming down from the HDU and needed to be kept separately for risk of infection. It gave us such peace of mind to know we were well looked after and not because of our own doing but because we knew God was reminding us that He was taking care of us.

We were transported by the porters - Martin carrying the bags, me with Teo in my arms. Being moved downstairs was a good sign. Finally, we would be able to have visitors in the private room. It was a humble space. One bed, one reclining chair, a TV, a window, a baby cot, a table and an en-suite shower. How thankful we were. It felt like a hotel after being surrounded by blue curtains, noisy beeps and chattering all night long. It was the first night we would be together as a three. We got settled and were handed over to the midwives on Larch Ward. Thank God for that private room.

LITTLE CLOTHES, HAPPY VISITORS

Martin and I had no reference for how our baby should look or feel as a newborn. She was our daughter and she was perfect. In between all this talk of my blood pressure, the baby doctors were monitoring her weight, her nappies and her general behaviour. At each point they were happy to see that she was feeding and making dirty nappies. She was a tiny thing - I had managed to buy tiny baby clothes during my nesting phase, but even those were far too big. I had three long sleeve vests that I was cycling round with leggings and enjoying the new joys of dressing this little wonder. Because she was so small, she felt the temperature change from warm and cosy to undressed and cold sharply. Her little cries were like music to my ears. Martin and I did everything together - nappy changes, clothes, sitting together and feeding. My heart was so full it could burst. Though the circumstances weren't ideal - having our little girl with us and learning to be her mummy and daddy was everything to us.

That first night in the private room was so special. I don't remember much sleep, but I do remember being cosied up together in the hospital bed. Martin and I together and Teodora on my chest or Martin's chest doing skin to skin. The midwife came to give me meds in the night and check she was feeding ok. I was concerned that she didn't like to be put down in her cot and was stirring a lot. There are a million signs in the hospital saying do not co-sleep with your baby. My instincts wanted her close to me, on my chest. She needed my warmth. The midwife reassured me the grunting was normal and that she was probably trying to say she needed cuddles. So I ignored those signs and let her sleep on my chest. She was much happier and so was I!

We had told our parents that we were moved to the private room. My parents were very excited that they would get to visit us the following day and Martin's parents on Sunday.

Saturday morning was a big day for us. One of the baby doctors from the NICU called Edmund had come to see us. He explained that if Teodora's head to toe check was fine and that her weight hadn't dropped more than 10% then she would be discharged and allowed to go home. It's normal for breastfed baby's weight to drop in the first few days as they adjust to feeding from their mums and not the amniotic fluid. We were so excited. It was just a case of my blood pressure normalising and then we could go home. We prayed and were hopeful and waited to be seen for the head to toe check. In the meantime, we were visited by photographers in the hospital and Teo had her first photoshoot! We had our first family photos together and the lady was sweet enough to disguise Teo's cannula so they weren't in the photos.

Soon afterwards, we organised for my parents to visit. I went for a shower whilst Martin got Teodora ready. I couldn't help but giggle when I saw how she was dressed. One of her white vest tops that had "Hello!" written in rainbow colours clipped over the top of grey leggings with butterflies with star printed socks and her white hat. I must defend my husband here and say he has great taste in clothes and dresses very well but in that moment I couldn't help but facepalm. I didn't want to disturb Teodora again - so we left her as she was.

Martin got a phone call - my parents were on the ward. It was time for Teodora to meet her Lola and Lolo (Filipino for grandma and grandad). I was so excited to see them, it felt like forever since that corridor and the chance meeting. I held her in my arms whilst Martin went to get them. I heard his laughter outside the door.

My mummy walked in first, on her tip toes with a balloon and daddy afterwards with a big gift bag. They were dressed perfectly and smelled amazing. I was touched to know they had dressed up for her. My parents always look their best and I also know the care and the time they take to present themselves. So it touched me to see them do this for Teodora. Martin presented their granddaughter to them.

Sacred. There is something very surreal about seeing how your parents love your child. You get a window into how they looked at you and carried you as their very own baby. You suddenly realise they were like you once, first time parents. Feeling the same things you felt. Even as I write this now, I cannot help but fight back tears. All those years I was a moody teenager or the times I didn't want to listen to them suddenly came back to me and I couldn't help but feel love and gratitude at their sacrifice and their love for me. Here they were holding our baby girl and the looks on their faces will be emblazoned in my heart always.

My daddy held her first, he spoke to her in Tagalog, he smiled and cooed over her. He laughed and giggled at her facial expressions. He fussed over her and wrapped her in a blanket. We tried to give her to mummy and she said, "Not yet, she is still so small." She was worried about hurting her to which daddy replied, "You cannot break them at this age, they are so malleable!" I watched my mummy hang back and let daddy have her. She never took her eyes off her. She was quiet and tender and watchful. I could see she was learning Teodora's face, taking her in. She was so happy. We took photos and enjoyed each others' company. They gave us cards and gifts. They didn't just get things for Teodora, they got things for us as parents. Always so generous. Most importantly, they brought us food! Hallelujah, home cooked Filipino food. I devoured the rice and tinola I had been craving for! Oh what a holy meal.

After a bit of coaxing mummy held Teo. I saw Teodora's face lean into her shoulder like she knew this was her Lola. A tender bond woven in moments. Mummy was there at our 16 week scan when the sonographer confirmed she was a baby girl. My mum was very quiet that day in the ultrasound room. Paul the sonographer was playing worship music and he prophesied that Teodora would be like John the Baptist, one who would tell her generation about Jesus. I hold all these things in my heart, that at every step of the way the Lord has been showing us that Teodora was always planned by Him.

The midwife interrupted us to let us know it was time for Teodora's head to toe check. Mummy and daddy got ready to leave and promised to visit again tomorrow. They were in love. I knew nothing would keep them away!

Martin and I wheeled the baby cot to the head to toe room. We prayed that all would be well. An older doctor did the relevant checks. He explained that a premature baby should have extra milk because they need to put on more weight. He said I would need to give formula as well as breast. I was adamant that I wanted to give her breast milk. He showed us the magic rocking technique. She started to wail at being handled and prodded and he picked her up in his skilled hands, looked her in the eyes and said, "No problem baby, what's wrong? Tell me…" and he motioned her up and down in a diagonal motion. She stopped crying and just looked at him. It was a move Martin would remember later in the night.

A FATHER'S JOY

I look back on those first few days and nights with a lump in my throat when I think of the love and rock I have in my husband. That Sunday, we waited eagerly for Martin's parents to come to visit their Teodora for the first time. To watch how she brought tears, laughter and tenderness to people's faces made us proud. But nothing was more tender to me than seeing Martin with his daughter. His baby girl.

Teo's arrival birthed in me a fierce love and strength. What I saw on Martin's face was a contentment and answer to deep desires that I knew he had ached for, for so long. What grace God gives, to use you as an answer to prayer. He has always been thoughtful and attentive, but to see this same care towards his girl makes me so proud of the man he is. He relished skin to skin, pulling her close to his face and nuzzling her nose, singing over her and drawing her close. He'd put her tiny frame on his legs and swaddle her in muslin blankets. He is not a man afraid to get his hands dirty or shy away from being there for us both.

After a quick phone call, Martin went to find his parents in the corridor. Teodora was wrapped in her blanket, all snuggly and warm. She was snoozing. I heard the familiar chunter of my father in-laws voice, excitement in his tone. Through the door, my loving in-laws. Martin was so happy to present his daughter to his parents. I sat back and let Martin re-tell our story and listened to him share his thoughts. Nana and Grandad sat on the bed with Teo between them, cooing and gazing at her. Nana had placed an instinctive hand on her chest and was speaking to her with the tenderness of a mother.

One thing about my in-laws that I absolutely adore, is their affirmation of praise for a job well done. They are prayerful and encouraging at every step. We were hoping that afternoon that I might be discharged seeing as Teodora had already been. We were waiting for the doctors to come and check on me. Martin went off with his dad to collect the car seat and a few bits from home. I stayed back with mum and Teodora.

My mother in-law is a wise and prayerful woman. Often in conversation with her, I find myself crying tears of release. She has a way of reminding me of the goodness and faithfulness of Jesus every time I speak with her. This time was no different as she shared with me her own experience of childbirth.

After they left, the three of us waited for news. By the evening, the doctors had come back to say I needed more monitoring. Another night in the hospital. Another night praying my blood pressure would normalise. Martin held my hand and reassured me we would be home soon enough.

DVT SOCKS AND DELAYED DISCHARGE

Monday morning, this was now our fifth day in the hospital. The familiar sound of midwives shifting from night duty to the day staff was evident in the corridor. The smell of toast and coffee was wafting down the corridor. I was thankful we were still in the private room. We had somehow managed sleep and I was feeling hopeful that today was the day to go home.

The four walls of the private room were beginning to feel claustrophobic. I was thankful for the early morning quiet of the hospital gardens. I had no idea what the outside world was doing. I was absorbed in a haze of newborn fuzziness and surreal hospital atmosphere. I had grown accustomed to the food lady who took my breakfast, lunch and dinner orders in the morning.

We had decided that Martin would continue his work whilst I was still in hospital seeing as I had the help of the midwives. So that day he prepared to head to school and tutoring. I was going to spend the day alone with Teodora. Surrounded by snacks, books, the remote control and my phone - I felt cosy. I meditated and prayed that by God's miraculous hand, I would be able to take my baby home today. I needed to have five readings of blood pressure that were within normal range. They had been amending my medication over the past five days. Today my doctor was called Doctor Tony. He liked oat biscuits. Helped himself to my packet which I thought was quite funny.

By 3pm, I was getting restless. Teodora has been good as gold, sleeping and feeding all morning and afternoon. Midwives came and went giving me meds and checking in on us periodically. I was still very sore after the c-section and was glad for the en-suite bathroom. I tried to walk around during the day to keep from feeling dizzy. I kept Martin up to date via WhatsApp and updated our friends who were eagerly waiting for the time they could come and visit.

I wasn't ready to see anyone outside the family just yet. I knew if I saw any of my friends, I would weep. I leaned into Jesus and gave my cares and worries to Him.

What is wrong with my body Lord? Heal my blood pressure. Please bring it down to normal levels. Lord when can we go home? Lord is there something wrong?

My prayers were silent worries that I knew He would understand. I could feel my body in battle mode. Yet every time I looked down into my arms, the smell and sweetness of this newborn gift calmed and stilled my heart in awe and wonder. I fully embraced the sentimental nature of my heart and let myself weep tears of thankfulness that she was finally here in my arms.

All those months wondering what she would look like, how she would feel, what I would feel and here she was.

This tiny and mighty miracle of God. I kept replaying the moments in the labour ward with Dr. James. She was ready to come. She didn't know worry, neither a sense of time. Here she was my lesson in blind trust - faith. She knew she would get food, warmth and love. Her instinct to find what she needed from me and her dad was strong. It what she was made for in her newborn state. I couldn't help but reflect on how this was a picture of how we ought to root for, seek out and long for God's love and provision. Trusting that He has absolutely everything we need.

My thoughts were interrupted by a hospital volunteer. It was time for another blood pressure check. I closed my eyes and breathed deeply. By this point I was directing them about which arm, which cuff and what side was best to take my blood pressure. Often the volunteer was different each time and I was trying not to get annoyed by it. She took three readings. Each one higher than the last. She kept telling me to calm down. Because that helps! She went to get another machine, but I already knew - it meant staying another night.

This time, she came back with Doctor Steph. Doctor Steph who came with a smile on her face and introduced herself properly. It makes all the difference when people treat you like a human being and talk to you as though you have a brain to understand what is going on. I will say, I only experienced one person in the hospital who treated me as though I didn't matter. The rest were very attentive and understanding.

Doctor Steph took my blood pressure herself. It was still too high. She said that she would come back and talk to me about what we would need to do. I explained that I had hoped to be going home that evening. It felt like she was gone for a long time. I called Martin who was on his way back to us. Teodora was asleep, peacefully unaware that her mummy was battling for peace.

She came back and sat on the bed by my left foot and explained that I would need to go back to the HDU (High Dependency Unit) for monitoring. She said I would have more attention there, they would be able to read my blood pressure more regularly than on that ward. She wanted to make sure that they got my medication correct. I began to cry. I was so frustrated. It felt like a blow. I was tired, I was frightened. I'll admit that now, it's a sobering thought when you realise you have no control over your body and what it's doing.

She took my hand and assured me, "We want to make sure that you get the right medication. They will be able to take

DVT SOCKS AND DELAYED DISCHARGE

greater care of you and get to a solution quicker. You will have a midwife assigned to you. There is less of that attention here so the HDU is better for you. I know you have been through a lot, an emergency c-section and an early baby. I know its not what you planned for. But you will be ok. Your body is realising she isn't inside you anymore and is just taking time to adjust."

I calmed down and thanked her. I felt God's kindness again through this nurturing doctor. I felt her rooting for me. I drew strength from her encouragement. I got my bags ready as they went to organise my transport for upstairs. Martin was on his way. Teodora was placed into my arms as I was wheeled back to the HDU.

It felt familiar. I recognised a lot of the midwives from a few days ago. Barbra was my midwife. She was there on Teodora's first night. She had helped me nurse. I didn't know then that she would become favourite midwife on the ward. She could see I was upset. I will never forget how she spoke even though I never said a word.

"Now mum, it's going to be alright. We will get you home. I know you want to be out of this place. We will get your blood pressure down. Just relax and let us take care of you. You focus on baby."

I smiled at her. She looked down at my bare legs.

"Where are your DVT socks?"

I was told I don't need to wear them because I walk around enough.

She looked at the midwife who was handing me over to her with disbelief.

"The patient has been walking around and doesn't need them," a sheepish reply from the Larch Ward midwife.

She looked over her glasses at me, "Now mum, we are going to look after you. You've had a major operation. You need to wear these socks. They will stop you from unnecessary clotting. I know it's hot, but it's for your own safety."

And with that - she pulled those DVT socks over my Filipino calves as though she was dressing a little girl. I was comforted in her firm approach. She reminded me of my mum. No nonsense. I like people like that.

There I was again, surrounded by royal blue curtains in the bay closest to the bathroom. This time I had a window. Teo was asleep next to me. She had no idea that this wasn't a normal environment for her - full of beeps and machine noise. Martin soon followed, his reassuring voice was greeting people in the corridor. He took my hand, prayed and blessed us. I was sorry to be sending him home to a flat by himself. I looked down at my DVT socks and felt sorry about my delayed discharge from the hospital.

DAY 6 - SCANS, WEIGHING SCALES AND THE NICU

Sleep was almost impossible on the HDU. You were only a few minutes from an emergency in the corridor. At any other time, I would relish listening to what was going on around me, listening into people's conversations and animated decisions. But that night, I was restless. I hadn't eaten dinner as I thought I was going home and left the dodgy hospital chicken chow mein unopened in the private room. I messaged my dad requesting some Filipino sustenance. I was sad that I couldn't have any visitors. By this point, I could feel the physical tiredness and uncertainty of when I was leaving start to cloud my peace. I was desperately fighting to stay in His presence and remain in God's promises. I would open my Bible and the words would feel blurry. The only thing, that kept me going was looking at my daughter's sweet face.

Having her with me was peace enough. She seemed to be

feeding a lot and no-one had really checked in on her since she had been discharged Sunday. Which I thought was a good thing. I managed to drift into a deep sleep between 5am and 6:30am. I woken by the lights going on and day shift midwives coming in noisily. Then the bustle of breakfast orders and medicine rounds about 7am made me start the day. I couldn't wait for 8am when I knew Martin would be allowed to see me.

My phone was a lifeline to the outside world. The signal in the HDU was very weak. The most I could do was text my friends and family. Their messages of encouragement and prayers kept me aware of being covered spiritually and that quickened my spirit.

Barbra said goodbye and I was handed over to Midi. A sweet Keralan midwife who we had met a few days before. Martin made friends with her very quickly. It seemed my blood pressure was still on the high side and so they were going to monitor me every three hours. I was under strict orders to stay in the bed, feed my baby and rest. That morning a community nurse came to say that she was going to do Teodora's 5 day check - a weight check. At the same time, I needed to go for a scan to check my bladder and kidneys were fine. Doctors weren't sure why my blood pressure wasn't going down. They usually expect blood pressure to normalise after three or four days. We were on Day 6.

DAY 6 - SCANS, WEIGHING SCALES AND THE NICU

Martin and I spent the morning with the curtains closed enjoying family time. Teodora was dressed in tiny baby clothes, white leggings and a turquoise long sleeve vest. It was my favourite thing to put her in at that moment as it almost fit her. She was very sleepy. We were taking photos and videos of her tiny feet and her little hands. Had we not been in the hospital, it would have felt as though we were at home simply enjoying each other's company.

The porter came to take me to the scan. Martin stayed with Teodora. Whilst I was being scanned, the community nurse came back to weigh Teodora after finding the weighing scale. I was cleared of any issues downstairs just as Martin rang to tell me I needed to come quickly.

Dr. Angus was there with Martin when I arrived.

Hello Doctor, good to see you again. Is everything alright?

Martin looked thoughtful. His face was serious. I got out of the wheelchair and sat on the bed. Teo was crying after being manhandled, undressed and dressed again. I picked her up and cuddled her close, telling her she was alright. Dr. Angus explained that during the weighing they noticed Teodora had red spots on her torso and that her weight had dropped further than 10% of her body weight. She was showing signs of jaundice and needed to be admitted to the NICU (Neonatal Intensive Care Unit). My face dropped. I had noticed one or two spots but didn't think anything of them.

Midi the midwife was there with us.

"But mum has been feeding baby all the time, every time I check on them she is feeding," Midi said.

"Because Teodora was premature, she needs more milk than mum can give at the moment. It's not uncommon for them to have jaundice. We will get the team to come and help you with feeding and learn how to use the pump," explained Dr. Angus.

My heart sank. My daughter was being separated from me into another ward. Martin asked the questions.

"What will need to happen?"

"She will need a dose of blue light therapy to combat the jaundice and we will insert a feeding tube to help her regain the weight she has lost. Babies this small respond really quickly to blue light therapy. We can take you round the NICU and show you the feeding room - I am not worried about her."

Dr. Angus had a way about him of delivering news without it feeling like it was a blow to the guts. Even though he wasn't worried, I was overwhelmed with the sudden changes.

Was my milk not enough? Why didn't I check the dots with someone sooner? How long will she be in the NICU?

He explained he would give me and Martin time to get her things ready and that they would bring her round as soon as possible. The NICU was on the same floor and I would be

DAY 6 - SCANS, WEIGHING SCALES AND THE NICU

able to see her at any time. That still didn't feel right. I sat on the bed and got her bag ready. Focused on what needed to be done. I could feel Martin's heart sinking next to me. This is the one thing he didn't want. He didn't want to be running between two wards. He didn't want to have to make choices about where to be and with whom. He wanted his girls home.

We didn't speak much as Dr. Angus took us down the corridor and into the NICU through the back entrance. He talked us through the different rooms and explained that as the babies make progress they are moved to different rooms. He brought us to the 1st room. A room with many windows, filled with natural light. I counted six incubator boxes. There were babies, each in their own incubator box or cot. The left corner box by the biggest window was for Teodora. He explained that she would be under the care of Nurse Crystal and Nurse Christina. Both Filipino nurses. There is something assuring about seeing your countrymen and knowing the level of care and love they put into their work. I introduced Teodora to her ates. Martin was very quiet. I took her into my arms and explained that she was going to be taken care of by these two ates. Inside I was weeping, but I had to be strong for her.

Stripping her down, I could see how many more dots there were. They placed an eye mask over her eyes and nodes to monitor her heart rate and oxygen levels on her body, hands and foot. She had to wear a special sock strap to keep the oxygen monitor in place. She got angry and started crying. I was secretly glad she put up a fight. The next part was the hardest to watch. They placed a feeding tube up her nose and she opened her mouth in a silent cry. My heart was breaking.

Vera Vera, the nurse in charge came over at the moment to introduce herself to me and Martin. She was warm and friendly and I could see from her face this was nothing new to her. She had a confidence about her that made me and Martin feel like Teodora was in good hands. She looked into the incubator and said, "There, there now Teodora, you are going to have a spa time now, a few hours of light therapy and you will feel so much better. Mummy and daddy are going to let you have some beauty treatment now."

It did make me smile. I turned to see Martin's face. He was fighting back his tears. I took his hand and we went outside. Nothing really prepares you to see your baby like that. I am sure it looks worse than it really is but it's not what you envisage. You pray for everything to go smoothly. You prepare as much as you can for possibly a few hours of pain in labour and then a peaceful time at home after a few days getting to know your baby. Basking in the glow of motherhood.

Nurse Crystal came out with a pump to show me how to pump my milk whilst Martin stayed to talk with Vera Vera. She led me to a little room with two pumping stations, a water station, steriliser and sink. She explained what I needed to do,

DAY 6 - SCANS, WEIGHING SCALES AND THE NICU

how to label my milk and where to bring it. They were arranging for a pump to be brought to me on the HDU as I was feeling so dizzy walking around the NICU. This was the furthest I had gone and walked in 6 days.

I found Martin making friends with the nurses in the room with Teodora. He was singing over her in worship and had struck up conversation with the nurse in charge of the room. Once again, we realised God's hand of provision and kindness in sending believers around our daughter. She encouraged Martin to sing loud enough for all the babies to hear. I was feeling tired but hopeful.

I was upset over leaving my baby, but having the task of pumping filled me with a sense of purpose. I had something I could do to help her whilst she had light therapy. Martin walked me back to the HDU and once again we called on the name of the Lord. We held each other and leaned into His words, that He would protect and take care of her, that He would heal her and bring strength to me. I prayed for Martin, yet again he was going home without us.

Midi came to check on me as it was nearly time for handover. Barbra was coming back. Midwives are amazing. Barbra came round the corner and her first question was, "Where's baby?" Midi explained what happened. Barbra saw my face, "Mum, it's going to be alright. NICU is a good place for her. They will look after her and you can focus on resting and getting better. Don't worry now mama, it's going to be ok."

I just nodded my head and swallowed the lump in my throat, she sat by me. I explained how tired and dizzy I felt. I hadn't slept properly for 6 days. I told her how noisy it was the night before and if I could get some proper sleep I knew it would help bring down my blood pressure. She said to leave it with her. She agreed sleep would make a lot of this seem better.

Barbra left me to pump my milk. All I could manage was a measly 10ml. No wonder my baby was hungry and lost weight. I looked at the 70ml bottle thinking, how was I supposed to fill that? I felt like a failure. It was a hard day indeed. I sighed heavily knowing that even that was a prayer to God.

Martin went to spend the night at my parents house. I didn't want him to go home to an empty house. Mummy text to tell me not to worry. She sounded relieved that Teo was in an incubator.

That night, Barbra was on guard. She hushed everyone that tried to disrupt the peace of the night. She even shut the door of the HDU, something I had never seen done all the time I had been there. I managed to sleep. A deep restful sleep.

DAY 7 - THE TURNING POINT

The next morning, the dawn light woke me up. The HDU was unusually quiet. I felt a difference in my mind and attitude.

This what it's like to wake up from a restful sleep. I was beginning to forget.

Barbra said goodbye and handed me over to another midwife. Midi was there again but she was assigned to someone else. My blood pressure was showing signs of lowering! Hallelujah! I had two lower readings. Praise the Lord. I felt hopeful but was not holding my breath.

Martin text to let me know he was bringing some *tinadtad* (my favourite Filipino dish of all time). My parents always know how to show their love. Food is a love language for me. He told me he would meet me in the NICU. I got myself ready to see my baby girl. I had prayed she had done better in the night. I felt well enough to have a shower and get out of hospital clothes and pajamas. I put on my jeans and floral t-shirt. I wanted to look good for Teodora.

The midwife cautioned me to rest for a few hours, my blood pressure still needed to be monitored every three hours so I mustn't miss my medication and reading times. I had to juggle the back and forth. So I waited till after breakfast, my 10am meds and blood pressure check before I headed over to her. Martin was already there.

Teodora had been moved to Room 2 - a good sign and was still on light therapy. My husband came to pick me up. I realised as soon as I stood up that I needed to take it easy with walking around. I was glad to have his arm to hold on to. We walked slowly to the entrance Dr. Angus showed us the day before. On the way, Martin explained that he had encountered another Filipino midwife who was talking about bottle feeding and dummies. She had no idea that Teodora was half Filipino and didn't really treat Martin like he knew anything. That all changed when she realised he was married to a Filipino.

When we got into the room, my baby girl was sleeping. Her face looked plumper and her tummy noticeably rounder. They had been feeding her round the clock with formula milk and the puny offerings of breast milk I had sent through via Barbra in the night. We had just missed the doctors rounds but Dr. Angus found us in the corridor and said he was happy with her progress. The spots had gone down and she was responding very well. That was our girl!

DAY 7 - THE TURNING POINT

We met nurse Jackie and she promptly came over to give us her opinion on bottle feeding, pacifiers and soothing Teodora when we weren't there. I knew she was trying to help, but I was adamant I wanted Teo to feed and to not have a dummy. We listened respectfully and then turned to focus on our girl. We were allowed to put our hands in the box after washing our hands and we could talk to her. She responded to our voices. I could feel my milk weighing on my chest. I decided it was time to pump. Martin stayed with Teo and I went to the pumping room.

Martin came to find me moments later, Dr Angus had said she no longer needed blue light therapy. Once again, we were rejoicing and giving praise to God. He answered prayers quickly for her. Nurse Jackie was asking for clothes so that they could dress her. I finished pumping and came back to the room. Underneath her incubator was a cupboard for Teo's things. It was nearly time for my next reading and medication. Martin walked me round and picked up some things she would need. He went straight back to her.

I told Midi the good news. She was so happy for us, but she also scolded me for not resting enough and said I needed to spend some time in bed. I just wanted to be with Teodora. I knew that I was on the mend, I could feel my energy returning. But I listened to Midi and got back into bed, had my meds, my readings done and tucked into some hospital macaroni and cheese - which wasn't half bad. Perhaps the news of Teo's improvements made everything taste better. I couldn't help but thank the Lord. I sent a text round to the family to update them and was met with their hoorays and joyful replies. They continued to pray for us.

The rest of the day was spent going between HDU and NICU. Martin and I took it in turns to sit with Teo. I was glad to see her dressed again. She still had the feeding tube in her nose, but she was looking so much happier. Martin had more stories of Nurse Jackie to tell and they were keeping us amused. She had shook her head at how ill fitting Teodora's clothes were and disappeared into the NICU supply of clothes. I came back to the NICU to find Teo in a pink knitted bonnet and blue knitted cardigan that fit her perfectly. She looked like a doll. I laughed but was grateful for Nurse Jackie's care. It felt as though this was a turning point. After a stressful day only 24 hours earlier, today seemed like a breeze.

I was still very dizzy and the c-section scar was sore. I realised after sitting with Teo and Martin another three hours had almost passed. Dinner was approaching and the doctors handover rounds would be soon. I went back to the HDU slowly that evening and resolved to be there for another night. It was joy enough to know I could walk across and be with her at any moment in the middle of the night if I so wished. Maybe tomorrow would be the day we could go home. Martin and I were hopeful.

When I got back to the HDU, there was a lot of discussion. A

DAY 7 - THE TURNING POINT

big group of midwives had gathered and Barbra was back for the night shift. I got back into bed and began dinner, prepared my pump for the evening feed. I could hear them arguing with doctors about the beds in the HDU. What I heard filled me with dread. Three new patients had arrived and were going to need to HDU space after their deliveries. They were asking the midwives to send patients down to the ward so that space could be made. I was silently praying it would not need to be me. I preferred the care and the attention of the HDU and more importantly it wasn't far from Teodora. The thought of being moved downstairs with the added challenge of moving around the hospital to get to her, knowing I was dizzy and sore was soul destroying.

I finished my dinner and waited. I could hear Barbra saying she was moving no-one and if they wanted to move patients the doctors would have to do it themselves. I liked her fighting spirit. I knew that my blood pressure was stabilising. I had had a couple of steady lowering readings throughout the day with only one spike. The footsteps of the doctors coming to the HDU and their voices brought an air of urgency into the room.

They came to my bay first. The three of them introduced themselves. A senior doctor and two others I had not encountered before. They looked tired and busy. Barbra explained why I was there and showed them my charts. I looked over at them expectantly. They began to explain what needed to happen.

"Based on your readings and your progress, we think it would be better to bring you downstairs to Larch Ward. We need to give this space to someone else and you are showing signs of stabilising," said the Senior Doctor.

I began to explain that this happened a few days ago, I was stabilising and then I went downstairs and medication wasn't given to me periodically and my blood pressure wasn't checked as regularly as it is up in the HDU. I aired my concerns that I didn't want the same thing to happen again. As soon as I explained that Teodora was in the NICU my voice began to break and hot tears rolled down my cheeks. I was annoyed at myself for crying. Because the real reason I didn't want to go downstairs was because it felt too far away from her. I knew my blood pressure was stabilising and it was good sign that they wanted to send me down. It was the last place you go before you can get discharged. But it didn't feel right without Teo.

One of the junior doctors stepped forward now, "I know mum, it's been a stressful few days for you and I understand your concerns, you've had an emergency c-section, high blood pressure, a premature baby who was a low birth weight, it's hard to sleep here, it's not what you expected... But you are getting better and your progress gives us confidence that you are doing much better. That's why we will send you downstairs. Someone can bring your milk to your baby so you

DAY 7 - THE TURNING POINT

don't have to go up and down too much. I know it's not the same level of care, but that's because we think you are doing much better."

She looked into my eyes and I felt seen and heard. She had obviously read my notes and taken the time to understand. I couldn't argue with that. They moved onto the next bay and began to tell the next person it was time to go downstairs. Barbra came to sit with me again. I looked at her and started crying.

"Now mama, you have to see this as positive. It's a good thing you are doing better. You are getting stronger and baby is getting stronger. Soon you will be able to go home. Don't worry, I will send you down last."

She made me laugh. She even took my blood pressure again and told me I will tell them you have spiked. I knew it was time to go back to Larch. This time there would be no private room or Teodora next to me. I began to pack and pumped my milk for the evening feed. I waited and waited for the porter. True to her word, Barbra sent me down last. I hugged and thanked her before leaving. God had sent a friend to me on that HDU.

LARCH WARD

I was wheeled to Room 11, to the end bay by the window on the right. There was no sight of trees from the window, only a white wall. Grim. I was surrounded by mums and their newborns. There I was, with a welcome to the world balloon and a bag of pajamas and clothes. The baby bed next to me was empty. My heart felt tired. I had had enough of feeling self pity.

One of my best friends texted me at that moment and I poured out my heart about what had just happened. She sent me a song and reminded me to worship God. We were nearly there. Martin had prayed for me before leaving and reminded me that angels were there to warfare on our behalf. Carrying the prayers of His people to God himself and bringing the comfort and answers back to us. I began to pray. I put together a list of songs on my Spotify.

Something happens when you take authority over your emotions. Yes there is a time to mourn, to cry, to laugh, to reflect and to ride the waves of what you feel. But at some point you have to realise they aren't to master you, but to serve you. I was fed up with not sleeping, with being in the hospital, with having a sense of uncertainty, it was time to rise up in my inner man and fight for my worship.

I had realised, I had been in a place of uncertainty and sorrow and if I stayed too long it may take over me. I don't know if you are a Spirit-filled, Bible-believing, Jesus-loving Christian or if you aren't sure what you believe. I am telling you between the frustration of the lights being on and hearing all the babies around me crying and not seeing Teodora, something in me snapped. It was time to rise up and fight in the Spirit.

I put on my headphones and began to worship. Took out my Bible and began to read promises over myself. I soaked in the presence of God who is always there to meet you at your point of need. Something hit me, a wave of strength. There are times when I meet with God and all I can do is weep and fall to my knees in gratitude. There are times when I feel His power fill me up on the inside and I shake and shiver from His touch. And there are times when I sense a light wash over me, like a peaceful stream that pours over the top of my head and flows through my body and I hear the clearest voice, a voice that I know on the inside of my heart is Jesus Himself, "This is how you fight your battles."

Let me explain, something happens when we worship. When we turn our eyes off of the reality of circumstances around us and choose to rise above them, we find that is the space where God operates. It's the place where He meets us. Face to face, gaze to gaze.

Yes there are times to pour out your cares and worries in tears of prayer, and times to mourn and allow your sorrow out in vulnerable submission at His feet. But in that moment, I felt the Lord come upon me, like a strong river. A strong peace. I saw my motherhood as a gift and this trial an opportunity to place all we went through in His hands as an offering of praise. I recounted the moments in the last 7 days where He had met us at our points of life and death, of uncertainty and pain, of numbness and tiredness. He had met us at every point. He was not about to disappoint us now.

> *I will lift up my eyes to the hills, from whence cometh my help? My help comes from the Lord who made Heaven and Earth.*
>
> ***Psalm 121:1***

I heard Him say, "Go and bring her milk and sing over her."

When you hear the Lord, you listen and obey. I pumped and for the first time, I managed 40ml for my daughter. The most I had ever made in one go. Praise the Lord. I got myself ready and braced myself for the walk to the corridor, from the corridor to the lift, from the lift to the NICU door, around the corner and into her room. With each step, though I felt dizzy, I prayerfully made my way to Teo.

I felt stronger by the time I reached her. She was sleeping soundly in her incubator by the viewing window.

She was wrapped tight in a blanket and her bed was slightly angled so that her feet were lower than her head. They told us that this helps with their breathing and circulation. I placed the labelled milk on top of her incubator and sang over her. My hand went to touch hers and she stirred. She knew I was there as I sang songs of deliverance over my girl. Songs to remind her that she was strong and full of life. She smiled and turned her head towards me. I cried happy tears. I knew it wouldn't be long now before we could go home. I knew that the Lord was turning the tide and we would see Him come through for us.

I left her with a new sense of patience for whatever lay ahead and I vowed in my heart to cherish everything that God would give us through this little girl. Already I could see the word being fulfilled that children are a blessing from the Lord.

I got back to my bed on Larch Ward, put my headphones in, put a towel over my eyes to block the light and fell asleep. A breakthrough night, a breakthrough sleep.

DAY 8 - A MOTHER'S COMFORT

I was aware of my blood pressure being taken as I slept but that didn't bother me. That morning, I was feeling like my old self. The me I was before the scar on my lower abdomen. It felt good to feel rested. Rest is such a gift from God. We cannot underestimate the power of a good night's sleep!

I had my toast and jam with tea, took a shower and messaged Martin. I couldn't wait to see him. Doctor Tony was around again and he was very happy to hear that my blood pressure was stabilising. Martin arrived when Doctor Tony was doing rounds. He explained that if I had 2 more good readings this morning and afternoon, he should be able to discharge me that same day. We were elated! He explained that I would need to carry on taking the medication at home till my GP was happy that I was ready to come off. I was also going to need injections in my thigh to ensure I didn't have blood clots. The midwife showed Martin how to do it so that he could help me at home.

We wanted to get upstairs to the doctors rounds so we could have a face to face update about when Teodora could come home. We were hopeful that we could all go together. We had decided that we didn't want our families to see Teodora in the blue light therapy box. Grandparents were allowed to visit but only one was allowed in the room at a time. Parents could come anytime 24/7.

That day, we told mum and dad they could come and see Teo. Told them that it might be home time for us. We managed to meet with the consultant for Teodora that morning. She had been moved from Room 2 to Room 3. Another miracle. I am convinced that the prayers the night before were heard. Our girl was making good progress and now their main concern was that she was putting on weight. Doc explained that she could only go home once the feeding tube came out and was gaining 150g a day. He explained that she would need to be combi-fed. A combination of formula and breast milk and that if we could take it in turns to feed her that would help. We would need some feeding support and to grow our confidence.

We spent that morning upstairs together with her. Nurse Jackie was there to teach Martin how to feed her from the bottle. We will always be thankful to her, she taught him how to feed our girl. I hadn't realised how he must have felt till afterwards not being able to be as practical with her as I had been in feeding from the breast. Teodora was so happy, her

DAY 8 - A MOTHER'S COMFORT

face was changing each day and you could see her colour and roundness improving. It was even noticeable after every feed how big her tummy got and how pink her cheeks were.

Those days in the NICU together were precious. I thank God he trained us around caring midwives, nurses and doctors. Had we not been there I probably would have given up on breastfeeding. I read up all about it before having Teo but the reality is a lot to take in. Without people around you to show you and advise you it is a very hard task. One thing I vowed in my heart was to persevere with breastfeeding, even if I couldn't carry my girl to term, I would do my best to feed her my milk. I was ecstatic that she was feeding well from both bottle and milk. I realised my girl was a hungry baby. The apple doesn't fall far from the tree.

That afternoon, we had the good news that Doctor Tony had signed my discharge papers. We just needed all the medication from the pharmacy. Mum and dad came to the NICU to visit Teo. They went in one by one to see her. My daddy held her hand and spoke to her. I could see the tears in his eyes. He spoke to her in Tagalog and told her to get strong. My mum did the same. Whilst they stayed with her I went to get my medication and my bags. Martin helped me to bring them upstairs so we could say goodbye to Teodora.

I was breaking on the inside to be going home without her. I went to meet mummy in the NICU and said a tearful goodbye to my girl. She took my hand and led me out. I held my tears till we got to the parent room. I sat down on the leather sofa and began to weep and wail. I had never felt such a fierce pain in my heart.

She should be coming home with me! She should still be in my tummy! This wasn't supposed to happen like this. I did everything I could to carry her well. Why did this happen? She's mine, she should be with me. I don't want to leave without her.

Everything I had been holding inside, came out in a deluge of angry tears and sadness. Martin tried to hold me and calm me down. I looked over at my mum through my tears and she came and hugged me. She comforted me and held me to her in only the way a mother could. She let me cry and then she said, "Come on, that's enough now. That's enough. Don't upset yourself. You know that this is what she needs. She was early and she needs the help. This is the best place for her and this is good for you. You need to regain your strength, you need to go home and sleep and then you can be with her. It's ok, it's all going to be ok. Yes, she should still be in you, but they can help her here. She will get strong. She is strong."

And I calmed down. Mummy's reassuring firm tone always does. She always knows what to do. She always knows how to comfort me. She might not have been the cuddliest or the most affectionate. She will say that herself, but she is so patient, so faithful, so steady and strong. That's my mum. I grew up hearing those words all the time, "that's enough now,

DAY 8 - A MOTHER'S COMFORT

don't upset yourself." My dad would also say those words to us. It was like a meditation for the Adamos House. You can be upset, but you don't stay upset. You need to remember you have a fighting spirit. That's what my parents brought me up to know. In that moment, those words were such a comfort.

Mum and dad made their way home and Martin brought me home. It was strange to take the car seat home without a baby in it. When we arrived back I had seen all Martin had done to prepare for his girls' return. The house was spotless, her next-t - me cot was there waiting next to my side of the bed. A space was made for her pram in the living room and everything I didn't manage to do before she came had been magically done by my wonderful Martin. The fridge was full of treats and snacks and he planned out meals and foods to keep me going. I was so thankful for my husband. He is a good man.

We were away from beeps and sounds of oxygen machines, the alarms and the buzzers of the hospital. I had forgotten what silence was like up here on the 9th floor. It felt like a weird dream being home without her. Like the past 8 days hadn't happened. The ache in my chest though told me otherwise. I realised how exhausted I was. Martin and I prayed and went to bed early. I was out like a light - dreaming of Teodora.

DAY 9 - BATTLE PLAN

Lines. The next morning there were lines and imprints all over my face and arms. It was one of those sleeps. You know the ones. Where you wake up feeling accomplished for sleeping so well you didn't move and the duvet made artwork on your face and body. I am not ashamed to say the dribble was celebratory.

We got ready for the hospital wanting to catch the doctors for Teodora's round. We meant business. Martin and I were back in tag team position. No longer living in separate places, but ready to strategize and bring our girl home.

I was excited during the Uber ride to the hospital. I couldn't wait to hold her, to smell her and hold her close to me. We got there just before the doctors and could see that they were briefing in the corridor outside one of the rooms. Vera Vera was around making parents feel comfortable.

Teodora was in a room with three other beautiful tiny but mighty babies. Martin being Martin, had already made friends with a couple closest to the window. They had been trying for a baby for more than 10 years, their son born 5 weeks early and a little bigger than Teodora. Another baby had been born at 26 weeks and had already been moved from another hospital to be at Newham. His mum was so encouraging. Her attitude and patience to wait for her son to be strong enough to come home spoke volumes to me. She was willing to sacrifice her sense of needing him close to keep him there and alive. If she could wait this past 6 weeks whilst he got stronger then I could wait as long as needed to take.

But Lord I hope it's not 6 weeks.

The last boy was early and had diabetes. All three beautiful boys fought to be here. All three sets of parents sitting by their babies cots cooing and attending to their children. We bonded in that room. We wished each other well and more importantly we blessed and prayed for each one.

Teodora seemed like the smallest in the room, but she was the loudest. Her cries made me proud. Nurse Jackie was there with us that day. Martin and I washed our hands and got settled around our darling baby. She was stirring. She'd just been changed and was all wrapped in her blue blanket. Our little miracle. She was no longer in an incubator, no longer covered by the huge warmer. She looked more like a newborn baby today, fresh in a swaddle and waiting to be picked up.

She still had the feeding tube in, the oxygen reader on her foot and wires to her chest to monitor her heart rate. But she was

DAY 9 - BATTLE PLAN

dressed and cosy. I picked up this tiny wonder and began to talk to her. Martin was taking photos. Nurse Jackie came over to discuss feeding. She was concerned about her putting on weight. As were we. She told me I needed to feed her as much as I could. In her Filipino way, she explained she wouldn't be able to go home unless she put on weight.

We were waiting for the doctors to come round to conduct the weigh in and discuss next steps. Martin and I were hopeful. We could see that she had been responding well to treatment and feeding.

When the doctors arrived, Vera Vera explained that only the baby being seen and their parents were allowed to be in the room. It felt very respectful to give each family and each baby that space. We waited our turn as they started with the youngest in the room - Mr 26 weeks.

I remember sitting outside the room with one of the other mums. She was crying because she wasn't able to nurse her son and was finding pumping really painful. I cried with her listening. I knew exactly her hurt.

Will I be able to give my child what they need? Am I enough for them?

Sometimes just listening and letting someone cry on your shoulder is enough. She didn't want to hear my encouragement or story. She just wanted to pour out her heart for a moment. That was fine. There would be more times like this. In the

NICU, you bond instantly with these parents. There's an unspoken bond of knowing you were all in the same boat, you didn't get the start you had hoped for. You are anxious about the one thing you don't want to utter out loud but the thought looms in the back of your mind - will my child make it?

Vera called us in. We stood by Teo's cot. We needed to undress her and have her placed on the weighing scale. The team introduced themselves and explained that they needed to see weight gain of about 150g per day for them to feel she was making good progress. My girl was cold. She hated being weighed. Her protest was strong and she wriggled in my hands. We held our breath watching the numbers, praying that they were enough.

Yay! She had gained that needed 150g.

Does this mean she can come home today?

The doctor looked at her charts, at us and then to Teodora.

"This all depends on her feeding. She's putting on weight because she's having milk through the tube. She needs to be able to nurse from you and the bottle. You can combi-feed her but it's important that the nurses can see she is feeding well. I think it's best we review it again in the morning. It's good she is putting on weight but we need to be confident about her feeding. She will not leave here with a feeding tube in her nose."

I could feel the slight disappointment from Martin beside me.

DAY 9 - BATTLE PLAN

We looked at each other and squeezed each other's hands. Martin was cradling Teo.

"How long would that take doctor? What's the process?"

"It's a case of her feeding. She is putting on weight. She is getting back to her birth weight which is a good thing. But really its up to you as parents and how confident you feel about her feeding. Spend today feeding her and being with her. Get support with nursing and them maybe you can room in and then go home."

What is rooming in?

Vera explained that before babies go home, they spend a night or two in the room-in space. A room made to look more like a home setting with a double bed, shower and television. It's a space where you spend time as a family with your child. It's almost like a test run before you go home to see what a night would be like nursing a premature baby. The nurse would weigh the baby at the beginning of room-in and not check on you again till the morning to weigh the baby to see how they have done in the night.

As teachers, planning and target setting is a game we know well. After talking with the team we felt we could come up with a plan. It wasn't what we wanted to hear first thing, but like Mr. 26 week's mum, we could learn to be patient. We wanted her strong and ready to come home. And more importantly, I wanted to know we could feed her enough. My

Filipino mum anxiety was strong inside me!

That morning, we learned how to combi-feed. Whilst I went to pump more milk, Nurse Jackie taught Martin how to feed Teo through a small 70ml bottle. It brought me great joy seeing my husband hold her tenderly and feed her. She was a hungry girl. At that time, we would have around 30-40ml through the feeding tube. The team had worked out how much she would need in order to gain the 150g per day. Each time she fed the nurse, myself or Martin updated the chart to write down how much she had had and what type of milk. At that moment, Teodora didn't seem to mind what milk she was having - just as long as she was having some.

Nurse Jackie was very happy with Martin's enthusiasm to feed his daughter. They had built a great rapport despite a funny start. The three of us were together again and everything was alright in the world. She was small but we could see her little character. Her little expressions seemed cheeky and playful. Her hands would startle and then frame her face like a vogue model. Everything she did made us laugh. I loved changing her. I didn't realise how much I would enjoy dressing my baby girl. I don't remember playing with baby dolls when I was little. My only memory was wrapping up a baby in "swaddling clothes" and pretending he was Jesus and putting on a blue cape pretending to be Mary. My mummy will tell you, I loved being outside, I wanted to wear shorts not dresses. I wanted to be climbing and running around or painting or playing

DAY 9 - BATTLE PLAN

teacher. But my daughter, my Teodora, was making me dream of little dresses, boots and socks. I had been looking up coloured bows and cute outfits. She had completely softened my heart.

After what seemed only 30 mins, Teodora was showing signs of being hungry once more. When you are that small your food goes through you so quickly. She wanted feeding every 30-40 minutes at times. I was happy to oblige. Nurse Jackie got me a screen and I got into position. Nothing felt more natural. She latched beautifully and we sunk into a warm cuddle. I began to cry, it had been two days since I had properly nursed her. She remembered who I was. She knew I was mummy. Her little hand rested on my breast and the soreness of my body didn't matter. I didn't mind having a broken body for her. The scar, the trauma of the past few days were far from me. I looked down at this little being. How powerfully this gentle girl could command such fierce love from us both. I never knew love like this before.

I will never forget that feed. It was as though she was pouring hope into me.

"Mummy, I'm going to be fine. We're going to be fine."

Martin sat there watching us both and we began to hatch a battle plan. We realised we didn't have any bottles, no formula milk, no steriliser. I hadn't planned on bottle feeding, I wanted to purely breastfeed. We made a list of things to go out and get. We decided we would have some lunch in the cafeteria and then make our way to Stratford for the necessary equipment. I wanted to be able to pump at home and bring milk in without too much worry.

Leaving Teodora in the careful hands of Nurse Jackie we went to implement our battle plan. We were determined to have everything in place to take care of Teodora. Martin was looking forward to sharing feeding and I was glad for the help. If she was to feed as often as she was doing, we would need to take it in turns.

THE MINEFIELD OF WESTFIELD

I am not a window shopper. Unless it's food, art materials or plants, I don't really find shopping that enjoyable. I love to have a list of what I need to get, go in and out and be done as quickly as possible. It's a good day when I can tick the list and get what I had envisioned.

That day felt like mayhem. Martin and I hadn't anticipated how mentally, emotionally and physically tired we were. The world had somehow continued to keep going whilst we lived in a bubble of blue curtains and hospital beeps. I had forgotten what it was like in a crowded shopping centre. We were overwhelmed by the sense of pace, of people's blissful unawareness of what we had been through. It was a sensory overload and something I had never experienced before. We went between two stores that were on opposite ends of the building and I could feel the pain of my scar starting to make me woozy. Maybe it was too much too soon. But we had managed to get what we needed.

We decided to head home and regain composure. He held my hand in the Uber and I held my womb to keep from feeling sore. I was due some pain medication soon enough.

That evening, I went back to the hospital to be with my girl. To hold her hand and snuggle. All I could see when I closed my eyes was Teodora. I had managed to use my new pump and was filled with purpose heading back to see her with my bag of milk. My supply was starting to increase.

She was asleep when I arrived and had just been fed by Nurse Jackie. I sat with her and watched her. I don't know for how long. I couldn't stare all night but I was aware that another good night's sleep would help my recovery and hers. The nurses switched over and I left my milk offering by her cot. I sang over her and prayed once more - blessing her to grow. Prophesying over her strength and peace, urging the angels to gather round her cot and watch over her.

Once again, I was going home without my baby. This time I was ready to be patient.

DAY 10 - ROOMING IN

Martin and I were there again before 10am waiting for the consultant team. Teodora had had an uneventful night. The nurses handed over and switched to day staff. The volunteers came round offering fruit to parents again. It was another day at Newham General's NICU.

Teodora was dressed and ready to meet her doctors. She was in Martin's arms when the doctors came round. Once more, she was weighed. It's amazing how quickly you can adapt to a new routine. This was now routine to us. Yet again, she had gained another 150g. This time the doctor checked her colour and alertness. She was wide awake and looking up at him with a sure, firm gaze.

"So you want to room in?" said the doc looking up at us.

Martin and I almost startled at his question. We had prepared ourselves for Teodora staying longer in the hospital. The doctor had read through the charts and nurses notes on Teodora's feeding and progress. He explained she was cleared of jaundice, she was making steady progress and that her weight was no longer a concern because he could see she was taking to combi-feeding well. He was offering us that room-in that night if we were ready. We were elated. Then the niggling hiss of doubt came into my mind.

Are we ready? What if something goes wrong? What if she loses weight again when she gets home?

So this is what it meant to be a mother. This sense of always thinking of risk and balance. It was as though Martin could read my thoughts. The doctor could see we needed to talk things through. They moved out of the room as Teodora was the last one to be seen that morning. My darling husband took my hand.

"Cheryl, let's room-in. She's ready and you are more than ready. You did remarkably yesterday. She is strong and full of life. She loves your milk. It's time to go home."

I looked into his kind face, his blue eyes. I love the kindness of his face. I could see him willing me to believe and have faith. What I have learned in our marriage, is that there are times he can see what I cannot. And when I am in a place of doubt and he is in a place of faith - I must lean into the fruitful truth of faith. I looked down at my girl stirring in her cot. How could I not want to take her home? Of course I did.

He took my hand and he prayed. He prayed then and there in front of the other families and babies in Room 3. I have always admired his boldness to be completely himself and

DAY 10 - ROOMING IN

completely sold out to Jesus wherever we are. It fills me with confidence anytime we are together and challenged me to do the same. I am covered by his confidence and hidden in it when I feel otherwise. He prayed thanksgiving for all that God had taken us through so far and for the wisdom and strength to do this next step. We committed Teodora into His hands once more. A prayer that we would pray everyday.

I began to pack Teodora's little clothes bag and gather all her accoutrements. She had somehow managed to fill two bags in a few short days. I was hopeful. Martin went to go and tell the team we were ready to room-in and I saw him shake the doctor's hand in the corridor. A father on a mission to get his girl home. A husband determined to take care of me. A man always ready to do what God convicted him to.

Vera Vera the head nurse came to say be ready in 10 minutes. It was all happening so quickly. Just like that, our girl was moving out of Room 3. I looked around at Teodora's three roommates and their parents. I had forgotten they were back in the room. I was sorry to be leaving them there. The mums were happy for us. They wished us well. I could see their complete joy in hearing our news. I went round and hugged each one and spoke a word of blessing over each of their families. I won't forget those parents, those babies. In such a hard place, there was so much hope in the atmosphere.

I picked up my baby girl, Martin held the bags and Vera Vera wheeled Teo's cot round to the rooming in space. We came out of Room 3, passing Room 2 and 1, waving at the nurses and doctors we had already been with in the past few days. They were glad to see us heading to the rooming-in space. We turned right down the corridor, closer towards the exit, passed the staffroom and the 3 critical care rooms. Rooms that I had not been in and not needed to be in. Rooms that had fewer babies in, lights turned down low and a nurse for each child. I silently prayed for each one as we walked passed. Keeping Teodora close to me, I couldn't help but thank the Lord that we didn't have to stay much longer.

We walked straight passed the first reception desk, passed the entrance door and to the end of the corridor. Vera Vera opened the door ahead of us. An actual bedroom. The room felt like a hotel room after all the hospital beds and spaces we had seen. There was a double bed, 3 seat sofa, arm chair and table, as well as an en-suite shower room. Bliss. Vera placed the cot next to the bed. She explained that she would hand us over to one of the nurses who would come and weight Teo and explain the rooming-in process.

She got us blankets and pillow covers, towels and a box of milk for Teodora. Martin was thanking her and talking to Vera. I was a little overwhelmed at how quickly we went from a clinical room to "hotel suite" in under 30 minutes. Vera said that they might remove the feeding tube by the morning if she fed well and put on more weight in the morning.

I placed Teo into her new space in the room. She began to cry

DAY 10 - ROOMING IN

and seemed uncomfortable. She was pulling at her face. Over the past 24 hours the tape holding her feed tube was starting to lose its stickiness. I knew she didn't like that thing. I wanted it out. I'm sure she did too. What she did next showed me her determination to enjoy rooming in.

"What's the matter princess? You aren't happy. You are going home soon. This will be your home for the night," uttered Vera.

With that, Teodora ripped the tape from her cheek and pulled the feeding tube out of her nose herself before any of us could help her. I was amazed. She cried. Tears of relief or frustration or both I wasn't sure. But I felt so proud. Here was my strong and full of life girl showing us she was ready.

"See mummy, she knows she's going home soon. She knows she doesn't need that feeding tube."

Martin and I laughed. Our girl was ready.

We called my parents and told them the good news. The next day was my mum's birthday. She was ecstatic. It felt like an answered prayer that Teo would be discharged for her birthday. Martin and I hadn't brought anything to the hospital with us that morning. We hadn't expected to be rooming in. He went home to get our pajamas and things for the night. More importantly her car seat so we could take her home the next day.

He got ready to go. Then there was just me and her. Bliss. She slept on my chest as I watched mindless day time television. She stirred, I fed her and then changed her. No-one came to check on us after Vera left us and handed us over to the nurses. They said they would weigh her in the evening. I enjoyed her. I cried happy tears. I was tired and happy. The room was hot but I didn't want to use the air-conditioning because I didn't want her to get too cold. My daughter was surprising me everyday. In my heart, I marvelled at how quickly she was changing, how quickly she responded to treatment and care. I thanked God. I thanked Him with all my heart. How grateful I was that she and I were alive to have these moments.

THE FIRST NIGHT

Martin wasn't gone long. He came armed and was ready with overnight things, snacks, food, baby clothes and a package for me. One of my best friends, Dulin, had thoughtfully sent lactation cookies in the post to help me with my supply. They were rich with oats and chocolate. Yum! My dad had also snuck in to bring us pansit (Filipino noodles) and rice. He was happily holding his granddaughter when Martin arrived.

After Teo's weigh in, the nurse gave Martin and me a piece of paper to log Teo's feeds and nappies throughout the night. We were to write down their timings and how frequent they were. After the door closed and evening fell upon the three of us, I realised how starkly different this felt. It hit me how "alone" we were with our daughter for the first time in ten days. There were no hospital machines in this room. The weight of responsibility hit me like a fear.

What if she stops breathing in the night? What if I don't wake up if she cries? Will we hear her? What do I do if I don't know what to do? What am I doing?

Once again - Martin was there to talk to and pour out my worries too. He squashed each one with the reminder that God gave us this baby and He was and is taking care of us. We lifted up the first night to the Lord and leaned into Him to guide us and surround us there in that room. We invited him into our parenthood and teach us to be the parents Teodora needed and not just what we thought was best.

We ate, I showered and we got ready for bed. I began a long night of nursing and finding the positions that would best suit whilst sitting on the bed. Martin wrote down every timing and every nappy. We took it in turns to get up and take care of Teodora. We drifted in and out of sleep. There was no cry we didn't hear. I think I lay there for most of the night listening to her sounds, getting familiar with her breath, her movements. She was pretty noisy.

The dawn met us and Teodora had found her way to sleeping on her daddy's chest somewhere in the night. She was happy there. Our first night was a success. The tiredness didn't matter. We were together for the first time since the private room on the Larch Ward.

DAY 11 - HOME AT LAST

The familiar sound of the food cart being wheeled down the corridor rattled in the distance and the mumblings of handover and night shift staff heading to their lockers came and went. A jolly, round worker came to take our food orders. It was good to see someone. We were beginning to think people had forgotten about us. In truth, it was 7am and the day in the hospital was getting into full swing.

We were happy. Teo was snoozing most of the time, we were passing the time cuddling her, changing her, feeding and singing to her. I loved watching Martin cuddle our girl and talk to her as if she understood everything he said. She'd smirk or smile when she heard us and it made us laugh. That morning a lady from the hearing department had come to check Teo's ears. She needed to be asleep when they checked her but both times she was wide awake. Everyone made comments at how alert she seemed and how strong she was.

By 11am the team of doctors had made their way round the

whole NICU and we heard a tap on the door. I was mid feed and Martin rushed to the door to protect my modesty. It was all very new for me and I was conscious of people looking over at us.

It was the moment of truth, Teodora's weigh in. Doc looked over our record keeping from the night, he was satisfied to hear that we were confident with feeding and changing her in the night. We got Teodora undressed and put her onto the scales - a full 1820g! Doc said it was up to us if we wanted to go home or spend another night rooming in but he was happy that she was on the upward trajectory. We said that we would discuss and let them know.

As they left the room and we dressed our frustrated daughter, I began to think again about whether or not we were ready. I voiced my concerns to Martin and once again he calmly pushed us towards going home. I went outside to the doctor to tell them we were ready to go. He was happy to write our discharge papers. All we had to do now was wait.

It wasn't till the afternoon that our papers had been written and signed. It felt like an age. We took the time to rest or in my case feel restless. We text our family and friends to let them know. It was Sunday the 9th of June - my mummy's birthday. I am sure the Lord has answered my mum's prayers that she wouldn't stay much longer in the NICU. We planned to head straight home and to get settled.

DAY 11 - HOME AT LAST

When the papers were finally in our hand, we said our goodbyes and thank yous to the nurses and doctors. Our girl was so small that she hardly fit into the car seat, even with the newborn insert. I had to bolster her up with blankets and a pillow. She seemed to snuggle in soundly. I wasn't anxious any longer. I couldn't wait to get my girl home and get on with enjoying the first few weeks together with our newborn baby.

I couldn't carry a thing, I was still walking slowly and aware of the soreness under my belly button. I filmed Teodora leaving the NICU and we made our way to the lift down to the ground. It felt strange to be leaving without a set of instructions or pamphlets of some kind. But I suppose it's not like that - you go home and get on with it.

The fresh air outside the hospital entrance was welcoming. I felt like I had been in the dark for a very long time, as though my eyes needed to adjust. Martin put the car seat and baby things on a nearby bench whilst we waited for the Uber to come and collect us. People were a few metres away smoking. Instantly, I wanted to shoo them away and blow their secondary smoke back into their direction. I wanted to cocoon her to me and keep her away from every germ.

Peace, be still. It is well.

I had to pray and speak to myself. We would be home soon enough. Martin had hailed the Uber and we were heading to the side of the pick up point to meet him when we heard two familiar voices behind us.

We turned to find Nigel and Liz, some friends from our church family, River Church - part of the army of people who had prayed for us whilst we were in the hospital. It was the first time we had seen anyone outside of our immediate family for nearly 3 weeks. Their smiles and their warmth set me off. I burst into tears as they congratulated us and gave us hugs. They spoke so sweetly and in hushed tones to ur sleeping Teo. They were the first to greet her and it felt right that we had seen our brother and sister in faith. I couldn't get any words out, I just cried tears of relief at seeing friends. Nigel gave me a big hug and said, "Well done."

Martin had to do the talking for us. I couldn't find the words to say anything coherent to them. I smiled and waved and got into the Uber, sitting with my dear Teodora. Finally, we were bringing her home. Home to the river, to the balcony and the barrier, where I had longed to hold her and show her the park and the trees. Home to her next to me cot and fresh clothes and teddies. We didn't know what the next few days and weeks would be like, but we were ready to enjoy being together and moving forward from our time in the hospital.

As we drove, I sat and held her hand and stared at this little wonder. Our gift from God - Teodora Joy Christin Adamos Noutch.

THE FOURTH TRIMESTER

Before Teodora was born, I soaked up every book, article and prayer devotional I could about motherhood, pregnancy, labour and the fourth trimester. I was a walking encyclopaedia of facts about breastfeeding, baby growth in the womb and watching my pregnancy app. I was obsessed with looking at fruit and vegetables saying, "that's how big baby is this week."

Even with all of that - nothing can prepare you for real life like living out real life. You can read testimonials from different mothers, watch videos and learn as much as you can. In the end your birth story is just that - your very own. It comes with no manual, no instructions, no small print - you become master of reading your child, learning about yourself and realising you were never meant to pressure yourself into controlling every variable of nature. It's impossible.

In the weeks and months that followed Teodora's birth, I went through many ups and downs, many low moments but also many unexplainable joyous times of simply being present and fully engaged in being with her. I suppose this part of the book is dedicated to sharing my experience of walking out my faith through the hard moments and processing all that happened with Jesus.

I write this knowing that there are many first time mums or mums who have been through similar to me, who believed God for a perfect story. You know, the ones where you believed for a quick labour, no c-section, out of the hospital quickly, lose the weight the next day and overnight magically become the perfect mum you see on social media or expect the same experience as your mum, your friend or relative. I read certain books that talked about claiming scriptures and telling God what you wanted. Whilst, I understand that prayer is powerful and speaking life over your situation as Biblical and Spirit-filled, I also know God is not a genie and for whatever mystery - life doesn't go the way you planned.

I can look back now and say - in my suffering, I drew closer to Jesus. In my questions and through my tears, I heard His promise to be with me. Here are a few lessons I learned and hope that they help you if you are a mummy who has experienced similarly. May you be greatly encouraged, your motherhood is a gift from Him and He knows better than you do why He gave you that child, that story and this journey.

THE GOODNESS OF GOD

The first week at home went by in a blur. I remember the only time we went out was to go for weigh-ins at the community midwife, watching television whilst feeding Teodora and being awake every hour in the night to feed. We were exhausted but we were happy. She was putting on weight and seemed very happy in her new environment.

I remember very clearly the day after coming home. We woke up, had breakfast and got dressed. Martin gave me some time to shower because nursing a baby in the summer months was sweaty stuff. I could smell my milk on every piece of clothing I wore and any time Teodora got close she was rooting for me. We had found a spot by the window on Martin's writing chair. It's a great chair. It used to be Martin's grandad's and had found its way into his possession. It was low enough that my feet touched the ground and wide enough to fit a feeding pillow around me whilst I nursed Teo. We sat there many times feeding and looking out the window.

That particular morning, a friend had send me a song, "The

Goodness of God." I hadn't heard it before. It was always my plan for my children to hear music and hear us singing and worshipping around the house even from the womb. There were many days where Martin and I would lay in bed praying over our unborn child and singing songs over her. That morning as I played that song, the words wrapped around the thanksgiving that I felt in my heart. Teodora was asleep in my arms by this point and I began to weep. Weeping tears of relief, release, joy and pain, sadness and joy all again.

He had led us through the night, through the fire, He was close like no other. In that moment, as I listened to the words of that song, I looked down at my little girl and marvelled at what the Lord had done.

Oh how easy it is to forget the faithfulness of God. Oh how the devil would love me to focus on how strong I was, or how me and Martin got through that without God's help. But the truth is, sitting in that chair that morning replaying what we had experienced in my mind, all I could see was how He helped us. From the moment I found out I was pregnant, to the gifts we received, the kindness of the doctors and nurses, the worshipping staff that surrounded her when she was born and how He got me through the darkest nights. I sat there and wept tears of thanks and praise.

The Bible says that He collects our tears in jars and knows each hair on our head. I looked down at my baby girl and promised I wouldn't forget God's kindness to us. I vowed to give my patience and my utmost love to take care of her and raise her in Jesus name.

Never stop being thankful for the big things and the little things. In times when I felt weary and exhausted from no sleep, irritated with my husband for not being a mind-reader and having no grace for myself - I put that song on. There were times when I didn't know how to pray because I was so tired. All I could really think of was complaint, but that song brought me to a place of thankfulness. Thankfulness is fuel for weary mothers in their fourth trimester - you will sure need to find the simple joys.

THE TIME SHE CHOKED ON MILK

We had begun to get into the swing of it. Martin woke up with me every time Teodora needed us in the night. He would change her nappy and I would go to feed. At other times, my parents who were nearby would come and spend an evening or a night to give our tired body's even 5 hours rest from feeding.

It was a Saturday evening, it had been over a month since we had seen anyone other than parents. I wasn't ready to let friends come and visit. This is very alien to me. I am a people person. People would say a classic extrovert, regaining energy from being around others. But after she was born, I couldn't risk her getting sick. I was hyper about germs and hand washing and keeping her warm. I knew that some of those thoughts were irrational but in my first time mum state, I was in protective overdrive. Martin was very patient and dutiful. He was my rock.

We had gone to the living room to feed to give Martin time to snooze. We were heading back to bed when I realised she needed a nappy change. The bedroom light was on and I went to take Teodora to the changing table. I got out the nappy, the wipes and laid her down. She began to cough violently and her eyes widened in shock. Milk started to erupt out of her nose and mouth. I screamed for Martin's help. I didn't know what to do. I tried to pick her up but she seemed to be choking. He jumped out of the bed and sat her up, patting her back. He tipped her forward and she vomited up loads of my milk.

"It's alright, she just choked a little. If it happens again, we just tip her forward. It's just a bit bigger than a spit up. She's alright."

He began to comfort her and I realised I had been holding my breath. I was scared. I ran to the bathroom to cry. I realised in that moment, I was completely afraid. In that split moment, all I could think was about her dying. I got on my knees and began to pray.

In that moment, I knew that I had allowed a spirit of fear to cause me to be anxious, worried and afraid of death. Many will tell you it is normal to feel all those things. But I say, those thoughts if not dealt with become a crippling mindset that steal your joy and your focus. I cried out to God. I knew that fear of Teodora dying was stopping me from allowing friends in, from going further than the midwives, stopping us from going to church and facing people. That fear was also trying to silence me from enjoying my newborn baby and owning the gift of motherhood.

I rose up in prayer and repented for allowing my unbelief and doubt stop me from living in faith in that moment. And like a new day, a clarity came to my mind. I knew what we needed to do. By this point, Martin came to find me after putting Teo back down to sleep.

"You ok, love?"

"Martin, tomorrow we are going to church. I am not going to let fear stop us."

VULNERABILITY MAKES YOU STRONGER

Getting ready for church that morning was surreal. I couldn't remember the last time I had taken time to get ready, to put on a dress and even look in the mirror. It had been over a month since seeing our church family. Having a shower and fixing my hair felt like a spa time. Motherhood truly makes you appreciate any moments you get by yourself.

We took the train. It was our first venture out as a family. Up until then the most we had done was travel to my parents' house to see my brother after he got back from the Philippines. I look back now and realise how cloudy my mind felt. It was a mixture of tiredness, medication and hormones rebalancing. I was fully myself learning to embrace this new role thrust upon me. I could recognise there were fears and insecurities bubbling to the surface of my thoughts and emotions. It would take some time for me to process them with the Lord. That morning was the beginning of building a lesson in vulnerability and testimony.

Arriving at the corner of Tant Avenue, I could feel myself take a deep breath. Martin had been chuntering and talking all the way, keeping me distracted. I felt a mixture of awe, gratitude and uneasiness. Teodora was safely cocooned in her baby pram. The list of no-nos I had reeled off to Martin were numerous.

No-one is allowed to touch her, Martin. We have to be careful of germs. No-one can carry her except us. We can use the baby carrier to keep her close. We must keep her warm. We'll stay at the back and just leave before the end to avoid a crowd. I don't want to be overwhelmed by people.

My gracious husband agreed and said, "We will do whatever is comfortable for you. Don't worry, I will look after you both."

Sometimes, when you leave things too long, they feel like an impossible mountain to get over. You build things up in your mind and a shadow comes along to cloud your judgement. I think that is how I felt about seeing people again. So much had happened. Where would I begin to even share or let people in again? Everything that happened felt so personal and so life-changing. Did every mother feel like this? All the books I read and articles I perused made out that with positive thinking you could overcome anything. I knew better. I knew I needed Jesus' help. Heading to church was our admittance of our need for Him in our lives.

Walking through the doors, we were met by smiles and greetings. There to greet us were Pawel and Monika, Polish missionaries, incredibly powerful and anointed people. People who had become great friends to us. Martin led the way and as soon as I saw them, I began to bawl. Monika held me and Pawel hugged me like a big bear. Dangus had also come to surround me. They simply spoke words of love and gladness in seeing us. I broke. Martin and Teodora had already gone inside to find a space at the back of the church. It felt as though walking through the church doors, I was surrounded instantly by Father, Son and Holy Spirit themselves. Instantly, I felt all that anxiety and worry about coming to church for the first time since having Teodora wash to the floor like chalk from a board out in the rain. Those thoughts were smokescreen lies trying to stop us from receiving a blessing that day.

After pulling myself together, they led me to Martin and Teodora and the seats he had saved us. People came by to say hello and kept a safe distance. They greeted Teo but didn't touch her. Martin didn't have to say anything. They all kept a respectful distance which calmed me even more. We felt safe. It was good to be in the house. The service started and we were lost in worship. I looked over at Martin crying tears of joy and relief, his daughter wrapped in his arms with a swaddle blanket over his shoulder. He looked so content. I sat there feeling the peace of God that passes all understanding.

As the service went on, I felt more and more of His strength replenishing us. The sung worship was stirring something new and reviving in us a determination to be strong in the Lord and the power of His might. I could hear the whispers of God speaking to me and looked at Martin. I could see the Spirit resting on him. It was a very special moment to know we were exactly where God needed us to be. I am always in awe when I sense these moments, that even in the trials and the testings, He is with us.

I don't remember specifically the message or words that were said that day, but something extraordinary happened. Martin and I often turn to each other and share what we are feeling spiritually. We both felt a sense of wanting to give thanks and give testimony for what God had done. Martin went to the front to testify of God's faithfulness and to present Teodora to the church. I was very happy to stay at the back where Martin had created our safe space. But as he walked forward, I felt a tug on my heart.

"Do you not want to tell of the goodness of God?"

I couldn't mistake the question in my heart. I knew I needed to allow all my fears and worries to be silenced by the power of testifying of God's goodness. Nothing is more powerful than giving thanks to God. It disables the voice of despair and sadness, it shifts the minds focus from self to God. I knew I

VULNERABILITY MAKES YOU STRONGER

needed to also say a few words. I knew I had to say something about silencing fear. Perhaps it would encourage someone else.

I went to join Martin at the front and stood with him and Teodora. He handed the microphone to me and I began to recount the sense of fear I had felt the night before and the lesson that God wanted me to learn. I spoke of God's goodness, spoke of how He led us through our darkest moment and how faithfully He had held our hand. That without God's help there would be no Teo, perhaps I would not be standing there that day. And I let the tears come and I allowed myself to be vulnerable to a whole church of people. And somehow in that vulnerability, in the breaking of my pride to show people I had been weak, the Lord gave me a fresh strength and a fresh perspective.

In the end, Martin and I ministered to people who needed prayer and breakthrough from feeling fear. I asked the Lord what to do because I had given Martin a list of things we weren't going to do. Praying for people would mean giving Teodora to someone. In the end the Lord told me to give Teodora to Dangus to hold. She was safe. I didn't need to worry about germs, bacteria and her being sick. The Lord had proved to me she was stronger than I thought - all through the hospital she was proving everyone wrong and ready to be in the world. I had to embrace the truth of what God was showing us about our tiny and mighty girl. As Martin laid

Teodora in Dangus' arms she began to cry - tears of thanksgiving, tears of peace. I marvelled at the thought that someone so tiny could have such an impact on someone already. Our girl was already being a blessing to people just by being who God made her to be.

By the end of the service, I couldn't help but laugh at myself. Martin laughed too. How irrational fears can be. I know some fears are legitimate, but in this new role of parenthood, I was sure we would have to deal with so many fears. With each one, we would need to lean into God. Lean into His promises that His gifts are life and life more abundant, that He takes care of those with young, that He comforts us just as a mother comforts her children. I had begun to understand, the best parents are the ones who realise they need the help. We aren't meant to be so in control that we become unteachable and set in our ways that we miss the blessing of transformation in Christ. This is why God says - children are a blessing from the Lord.

We went home that afternoon with light hearts, treasuring what the Lord had done for our family that day.

DON'T LET YOUR MIND WANDER INTO LIES

One of the hardest parts of this journey has been dealing with the trauma of what happened. I didn't even want to admit that it was traumatic, but looking back my body and mind had been through something I hadn't expected. No-one can plan for that. I would love to tell you that after a few weeks I was back to my old self and ready to face the world. I treasured every moment with Teodora. Her smells, her smiles, her little movements. Every single moment together as a three was precious. Martin was working part time in a school 2 days a week and working some evenings tutoring. After 2 weeks of paternity leave, he was still mostly with us 5 days a week. Even in that timing, the Lord had made a way for us to have an extended time together. In the end we had the first 3 months together and it was perfect.

My mum and dad would come on the days that Martin was at work. Teodora and I spent time out in the park walking, sitting on the bench. She would sleep on my chest and snooze there happily whilst I rested and scrolled through memes. There was no routine in those three months, it was all about getting to know each other and accepting that tired and sleep deprived was the new normal. She was a very easy baby. I couldn't complain, nor did I want to. She was our little miracle.

But I realised that in slowing down into a new pace of life, time and quiet had led to many moments of reliving our experience. In between midwife appointments, weigh-ins and our daily walks, my mind had a lot of time to think. I think many first time mums would say they experience a sense of "losing self" or grieving the woman you used to be. I understood in theory that life would be different but I was beginning to feel resentment. An ugly feeling. I imagine it to be a stench, like something in the bin quietly rotting away until you realise you need to take the rubbish out.

I was resentful of the fact that my loving, supportive husband could go out to work and have time to himself. I was annoyed at the fact that I had to wait till someone was with me before I could really relax into a shower without feeling guilty for having time for myself. I was frustrated that I had no time to even read or pray, I always felt I needed to be on high alert to attend to my daughters needs. I knew this was a period of adjustment but it was hard. I wanted to be someone who could take it all in my stride, but again I knew this was something I needed the Lord's help with. I didn't know how to talk about how I felt without sounding ungrateful or guilty. Every time, I looked down at my little girl nursing or sleeping next to me, those feelings went away. How could I feel this way when I had the most amazing gift of my life here in the world and I got to be her mummy?

Coupled with all of this was self pity. Another ugly sense of myself. I was well aware I was dwelling on things I could not change. But there were questions I had. Answers I needed.

Why did this happen to us? Was there anything I could have done in pregnancy to stop this happening? Did I do something to upset God? Was He punishing me?

Sense came in the form of my mother in law, Anna. I will never forget how she counselled some of my fears and worries in those early days. She sat me on the bed after I'd changed Teo and spoke right into my heart. After a tearful exchange of me opening up all that I had been pondering, she looked me in the eye and said, "Cheryl, don't go there. Don't even go there. Those are lies. You know that. Teo's timing was the Lord's timing. He makes no mistakes. You were ready. The enemy wanted to steal, to kill and destroy but God is faithful. Remember the Lord is faithful. He wrote the story. Don't let the enemy steal your testimony. You did nothing wrong. We will never know why some things happen and even in that we have to trust the Lord. He always has our best interests at heart. Keep trusting Him."

I need reminders, I need strong, godly people to come alongside me and encourage me when I feel weak. Once again, I was reminded to arm myself with praise and thankfulness, to keep my heart in a place of focusing on who truly mattered, God Himself. God taking care of us.

DYING TO SELF

We all need help. Social media and the world paints a pressure cooker of a picture, where women and mothers need to be able to juggle and have it all and do it all looking fabulous. You know the kind - the super organised mum with perfectly manicured Muji drawers, pantries with labels, highlighted schedules, routines timed down to the nearest millisecond. Able to find time to have dinner with their girlfriends and have weekly beauty treatments, not forgetting juggling businesses, careers and entrepreneurial pursuits. And according to Instagram have perfect marriages and date nights. It's an unrealistic goal. Sadly, even Christian circles can paint this picture and very few words are said about growing more Christlike through suffering.

Isn't pregnancy and motherhood also about sacrifice and suffering? There is a victory in proclaiming that truth. Those feelings of resentment and self-pity are once again lies that prevent us from operating in a place of victorious motherhood. The place where the redeemed, restoring and reconciling power of Christ can partner with our weakness and transform us to be more like Him. Did he not know what it meant to suffer? Dying on the cross and sacrificing His body for all man's sin?

One particular lesson I am learning to take hold of each day in becoming a mum is to embrace dying to self. Trying to show the world you are keeping it all together is a pressure we as mothers do not need. It can be a subtle pride that stops us from really connecting with other women who may be feeling similar. I am not the same woman I was before I had my daughter - for this I am so grateful. We have to be kind to ourselves. This is more than self-care, it's about dying to self.

What do I mean? Are you willing to let your expectations, your hopes, your dreams, your desires to die and entrust them to God? I never dreamed I would write a book of our experience and through it receive so much healing and release. If I choose to fight for the truth that in Christ I have everything that I need, then I can receive from Him more than I can imagine and ask. If I need strength for the day, wisdom for how to raise my family, more grace and love towards my husband - then I know where I can run. If I think, I can do these things myself by re-organising my schedule and telling myself I can push harder and do more, then I miss the place of rest where God can speak to my deepest heart desires.

Another tiring morning led me to pick up the phone to my mother-in-law, I knew that I needed to deal with the resentment and bitter thoughts that were trying to weave their way into my heart. I was tired of the mundane everyday tasks and not feeling stimulated. Baby classes and sensory groups seemed to be my only social jaunt and whilst it was cute and fun, I wasn't in the mood to be making new friends and having small talk.

Once again, wisdom spoke, "This is about dying to self, Cheryl. Your husband needs you, your daughter needs you. Take heart, God knows everything you need. I have been praying for you. I know what it's like, it can feel all too much at times but remember to be thankful. Don't let pride come between you and Martin. Your marriage comes before motherhood. He is faithful."

Once again, I needed that reminder to look up. Everything we need is found in Christ. My sense of self would have me believe I was the most important person in our family, that everyone needed to think more carefully about me, I was the one who had been through so much. Boohoo! Hoo! What a debilitating way of thinking. What a stinking lie! Once more I needed to admit, I was partnering with my weakness. Partnering with a selfish, worldly way of thinking that bore no fruit but bitterness. Pride reared its ugly head again.

We build so many walls that teach us independence is powerful, being strong is successful and asking for help is weak. Perhaps, Teodora coming the way she did was God's way of showing me how much I needed to live out the truth of the gospel. I have prayed so many times that I may know

Christ and know the mighty power that raised Him from the dead, I have prayed that I may know His suffering so that I would know the power of resurrection (Philippians 3: 10-11). Be careful how you pray!

The gospel can be lived out even in our daily lives. It's not just about big crusades and evangelising on the streets. It's also about letting pride die in your marriage so that Christ can be displayed in your relationship. It's asking for help and admitting you need more support with tasks you once took for granted like cooking dinner and hanging the washing. It's admitting that you do not have all the answers about how to raise your child, but you are willing to turn to God who has all the answers. The gospel is lived out in humility in our homes. The gift of motherhood is teaching me so much about how selfish I have been and how willing Christ is to help me change.

Dying to self is a gift. Admitting imperfection in His presence and accepting He is a perfect God willing to love us through our ugliest moments is something I didn't anticipate in this journey. It's beautiful and crushing but worth fighting for.

"THAT C-SECTION SAVED OUR LIVES CHERYL!"

When Teodora was 4 months old, we travelled to a weekend retreat. It was our first holiday as a family set in the beautiful grounds of Ashburnham. Martin and I had been to so many Renewal weekends on day passes, but this was our first retreat. I was so excited at the thought of having time to worship in the countryside with our daughter. I was looking for some much needed relief and maybe the Lord would clear more of the niggling thoughts that had been plaguing me. I was feeling restless inside.

God had done so much already. Teodora was growing beautifully, she was doing so well. We had been switched from the community midwife to the health visitor. Instead of going for weigh-ins every 3 days, where we went to monthly weigh-ins. She was filling out her tiny frame and growing rolls upon rolls of pure breast milk. Martin reminded me over and over again that her weight gain was because of me committing to nursing her. I felt so proud of that. I might not have been able to push, but I was determined to feed her on demand. Even if it hurt.

From the moment we arrived on the green of Ashburnham's lush grounds, I was aching to have some time to myself. We got settled in our little ensuite room. Packing for a 4-month old was no easy feat. As well as her own bag, she needed a changing bag, her next-to-me cot, many options for clothing depending on the weather. I had never known such a mental load before. How many nappies would I need for 3 days, plus extra? What were the bathroom facilities like? We needed the pram and the baby carrier, the car seat and everything I could possibly think of to keep her comfortable. Oh Lord, what an experience travelling with a little one is like. Poor Martin had to do a lot of lifting.

We arrived late on Friday evening and there was just enough food left for us to have dinner. Praise God. We were hungry. Teodora travelled so well, she slept most of the way and was alert and ready to meet new people. She was smiling and winning everyone over with her chubby cheeks. We decided that we would not try to push too hard to attend every formal meeting, but take our time and go at our own pace. That evening we decided to go back to the room and just spend the evening together as a three. Our lovely Teo was beginning to enjoy our songs and showing us she was listening with coos and smiles and kicks. We didn't want to miss that.

By around 9pm, she was fast asleep next to me and I could feel the tug to get to the outdoor tent to catch the end of a worship meeting. I wanted to dedicate the weekend to the Lord and just get my head and heart in a place ready to listen. Martin stayed with Teodora and snoozed after the long drive down and I found myself walking down a garden path to the sound of a distant voice on the microphone.

The lights of the tent were welcoming and the space was mostly full. I found a seat at the back and sat down, they were about to end the meeting. Someone was up on the piano and they were preparing to offer prayer to anyone in response. I saw some familiar faces and friends in the crowd that we had come to know over the years.

I don't remember what the altar call was for, but I remember running to the front. I knew I just needed to surrender the heaviness, the tiredness and the weariness of my heart to the Lord. I have no qualms in saying, I am not ashamed to get on my face to seek God, bend my knees and pray. I know my limitations and I embrace the correction and love of God at every opportunity. I never want to miss what He wants to say to me. This evening was no different.

The worship team began to sing, a song I hadn't heard since that night. The night she was born. The familiar piano line begun and the lyrics flooded my heart - Waymaker.

My knees buckled under the weight of the words that I had

last heard when Teodora was born. I hadn't listened to this song, I hadn't allowed myself to listen to my "birthing playlist" because it was too hard. I suppose it triggered something deep in me. I was a mess, a heap of tears on the floor, crying loudly, I didn't care who heard. I was there to meet with God and exchange every wrong thinking I felt, every hurt and pain and sorrow I felt about Teodora's delivery that weekend. It was something that I found hard to deal with.

I am used to seeing myself as strong and a "get on with it person". I hurt and I have my moments, but my mummy always taught me to have a fighting spirit. You don't dwell in a place of hurt or pain, you don't stay there. You stay in a place of joy and encouragement. But this felt so different. I had been in this place of mourning, of shame and sorrow for months. My heart began to soften in that place of worship and for the first time, I allowed myself to surrender how I was feeling. I didn't want to feel this way anymore. I didn't want to try and "fix it" with my own remedy or strength. God knew it hadn't worked so far.

That night, a lady I do not know came to me at the end and said that she saw a huge cloud and that God wanted to blow it away. She told me, it was time to sing again, to trust God again and receive a fresh grace for the season ahead. Those words deeply encouraged me as I walked back teary-eyed to the room.

One thing I love about the countryside is how dark the night is. There is no light pollution. Heading back to our room, I knew I would sleep so soundly.

The next morning, we needed to wake Teodora up to get to breakfast in time. That's how good her sleep was. The country air and dark night was good for all three of us. We woke up feeling refreshed. The walls were a little thin and you could hear people coming and going to and from their rooms, but that didn't bother us too much. We didn't need the next-to-me cot, she spent the night sleeping cuddled up to my armpit - a place she had learned to nestle and love.

We were there amongst family. It was the first time a lot of our Renewal family were meeting Teodora and she greeted them all with smiles and alert stares. Martin and I managed breakfast together whilst our good friend Scott scooped Teo in his arms. She didn't seem to mind. It was lovely to feel taken care of. Small kindnesses like these make me think of the Lord and the simplicity of finding His provision in seemingly everyday moments. Little kindnesses.

After breakfast, we went to our first session. We sat and listened to teaching and enjoyed worshipping together most of all. There were flag worshippers and spaces at the back of the tent to move freely. Martin enjoyed having Teodora facing outwards in the baby carrier whilst he sang and danced. I enjoyed being in that environment of free worship.

There was a moment where we had to get together and pray

with people around us. I had already been feeling throughout the meeting that I wanted to shout and let out my praise. I was pacing up and down the back of the tent, wrestling with the idea of making so much noise. I know it is good to obey when you feel the Spirit of God stir you, but there are times when your human mind wants to fight your inner man. The moment came, the speaker explained that he had also felt the urge to shout and began to recall the story of Joshua and the Israelites walking the walls of Jericho for seven days and on the seventh day letting out an almighty shout which broke the walls down. Hallelujah - I knew the Lord would be gracious to give me space to do what He asked.

As we pressed in through prayer, I felt that burning in my heart to lean into God. To allow myself to let go. I let out an almighty cry, others around me did the same. I felt the Lord speak right to me.

Cry and shout, take back your shout of labour. Birth in the Spirit, birth in the Spirit.

I cannot explain to you how it felt to hear the Lord tell me to take back my shout. I remembered the words from the lady last night, who told me it was time to sing again. I hadn't realised that in the months that followed Teo's birth, I had grown silent. I had allowed my voice to be stifled. I cried and shouted with all my might. Then we were instructed to gather in threes and pray with people. I ended up with two other women - Toni and Crystal. We were weeping, praying and crying over each other.

"I feel like we are birthing something new for ourselves and for our nation. It's the ninth month of the year and the ninth month is when women give birth. I feel this prayer is significant as we are three women praying."

That is more than a coincidence. How would she know I was there praying and sensing similar thoughts about birthing and dealing with something so personal? Only the Spirit of God would do that. I felt that God had hand picked those women to pray with me. I felt so loved and encouraged by God Himself at that moment. How could I forget His goodness? How could I forget His faithfulness?

I couldn't say much as we stood in that prayer circle, but I knew I wanted to speak to Crystal during lunch. So that's what I did. In the lunch line, I found myself next to her and her mother. I began to share what God had said. She saw Teodora and I explained that she was six weeks early. I began to recount my story of the night she was born and she began to speak.

"You had an emergency c-section, you had to be injected with magnesium and the painful leg steroid. You could have died that night, your baby was at risk wasn't she?"

I was dumbfounded. *How did she know? How could she know?* She saw the shock on my face.

"I know Cheryl, because fifteen years ago, that was me. I had preeclampsia. I was in the hospital in exactly your position. I had to sign a waiver that said if something happened they could remove my womb from me. I remember saying, my God will look after me. Do you see that young man over there? That is my son. He was also six weeks early, he was a tiny thing. Look at him now, he's bigger than me. I know that God has such a special plan for his life and the devil wanted so much to take him from me and not let him live. Our children are a gift from God. God had other plans."

I hadn't said a word. I fought back hot, salty tears.

"Cheryl, when we have a chance, I would love to pray for you, your daughter and husband. I will even ask my son to pray for your daughter. But I want to say this to you. That c-section saved our lives, Cheryl. God used that c-section to save your life."

There it was. The lie that was looking me blind in the face. The lie that having a c-section was my source of shame. That I couldn't push, I couldn't carry her, I wasn't a proper mother because I didn't labour naturally. God sent Crystal to speak right into my heart and break the veil over my mind and eyes. I hadn't even realised, I had cursed myself in thinking those things. I had disengaged with my body somehow and harboured unforgiveness towards myself. The devil had worked overtime to silence me, blind me and bind me. To try and rob me of my joy from God.

"When you face your own mortality, you become so much closer to God. You recognise how much of a gift life truly is," she said.

And then, she just held me. Hugged me and wiped her own tears as we cried. Bonded over our shared experience. How good it felt to be known, to be understood without even having to say a word. Once again the Lord was making clear to me He was seeing, hearing and understanding everything in my heart. Little kindnesses.

IT TAKES A VILLAGE

I didn't want to write this book without saying a word about what it takes to raise a family. The Western world has a lot to answer for when it comes to projecting a culture of success that says, "I build this empire myself" and "I did it my way." The truth is, we all need help. We all need support. One of the ugliest things I have seen amongst women is a spirit of comparison, competition and falsehood.

Comparison means you don't share what's really going on for fear of judgement. Instead a subtle one-upmanship can permeate even the closest of friendships. Competition cries "Look at how well I am doing!" Whilst silently, behind closed doors mums are insecure about every detail of life from how well their child is sleeping, to their development, their weaning and their weight. The enemy tries so hard to cause women to compete against each other. It's something we all have to guard against.

I am afraid to say I have seen this amongst mothers. It's there in the questions, "How much did he weigh?" "Is she sleeping through the night?" "My daughter can say 50 words and she's not even 13 months old." Instead of celebrating the unique character of each child, we pit them against each other as a tally of success in our motherhood. Ouch!

The truth is - it takes a village. It takes friendship, vulnerability and humility to truly raise a family. I look back on everything we have been through as a young family raising one child and see all the generosity and love poured into our daughter from family, friends, church and colleagues.

In my first few weeks of motherhood I needed my mum and my family more than ever. I needed the help of my husband to chop my food whilst I breastfed at the table. I needed best friends to come over and make meals, hold the baby whilst I showered and had a cup of tea. I needed my daddy and brother to come with me to doctor's appointments and immunisations because I was still weak from the c-section. I needed to ask for help.

The village around us were amazing. They were a beacon of God's love and kindness once more in the form of cots, prams, changing tables, clothes, nappies, frozen meals, toys, online food orders… the list was endless. The kindness we received was miraculous. Once again the Lord was undoing the concerns and fears I had about provision through the people around us. If you ever doubt you are loved and cared for, see what happens when you need help. The response will astound you! You are more loved and cherished than you can fully grasp!

When I look around our flat, I see the pram and the changing table our godparents gave us, the car seat our close friends passed onto us. Our daughter is wearing clothes lovingly picked and given to her by various friends and family. The knitwear from nana is particularly beautiful. My own parents never stop giving to her and through all these people we receive the Lord's blessing. They give their time and their support so readily and we are so grateful for them. I won't forget those early days and weeks when Martin and I just couldn't get Teo to sleep. My parents would come in the evenings and just love on her, patiently rock her, try out different positions to get her to sleep. They were training her and us as parents in their gentle and loving way. They would send me and Martin to bed so that we could have a few hours rest. Some nights I'd wake up with a start realising we had slept till three in the morning and my parents would be up in the living room just singing to her and helping her sleep. Their patience and love is such a lesson to us.

At every point of pregnancy before I could even take out my wallet to buy the things that I had planned to give her someone came and said, I want to give this to you. These are huge blessings! Before we even conceived I had many fears about how we would provide for children. It was one of the things that held us back. But time and time again God showed up. So I want to encourage those of you who are worried about provision for your families, trust in the Lord!

The village included four of my friends who were pregnant at the same time as me. It was a special journey walking through similar experiences together, meeting up and sharing our hopes and fears, praying for one another and rejoicing with one another when our babies came. One of those friends in particular is my dear sister in Christ, Afia, who not only led me to Jesus when I was nineteen years old, but has continued to be a solid sister and best friend over the years. We have spent hours voicenoting our prayers, our cares, our woes, laughter and frustrations! Truly you need members of your village who can keep you laughing. They are the ones who can hold a mirror up to your fears and irrational thoughts and tell you about yourself. We all need that in life - not only motherhood! The village of fellow mothers around me are a shining light of grace and understanding. They are the ones who bring your favourite meal and hold the baby to give your arms a rest or randomly bring you a mango because they know you like it.

The village has also been an army of prayer warriors who rallied around us that night and prayed for our safe delivery, for Martin as head of the house and for our dear daughter. I will never forget how my best friend Ayanna rallied her church to pray. The voice notes, songs and encouragement we received whilst we were in the hospital were a tonic to me. They were precious messages of hope and I felt so secure knowing the Lord was using all these beautiful people to cover us in prayers.

Our own church family at River and my family at The Revival Church were such warriors gathering to pray, send scriptures and messages too. They continue to be such solid rocks to our village and our family. We cannot say we are raising our families on our own. We are raising this daughter on the shoulder of a praying, encouraging, championing, strong and generous village who honour us with such kindness, love and strength.

There were days when I forget that there are people so ready and willing to help. Mothers - do not isolate yourselves, reach out to your village. They are a lifeline and a gift from God. The Lord uses them to strengthen you when you least expect and even when you don't feel like seeing them.

FORGIVENESS AND MILESTONES

The truth is, I would be here for volumes writing down every little kindness I have experienced from the Lord over this past year. I want to do this story justice and tell it as true as I can, to give glory to God and to be honest as a believer about what we experienced. I know the promises of God, I love His word and I love to worship.

When Jesus talks about giving us life and life more abundantly, I don't imagine we think about our suffering as part of that abundance. But in this past year, I can say I have had more abundance and more true living than I have in my previous thirty-three years. I don't say that lightly. It's more than just blessing, success and feeling content - its learning to embrace the weakness, lean into Him through the hurts, the worries, the cares and truly receive the revelation of rest, of grace, of His rich treasure and knowledge beyond human understanding.

I do not claim to have it all locked down. I fail more than I win and that is ok. I would rather have a life where I learned to tumble and fall in His presence receiving His correction than a life of bumbling along from week to week with a shallow religion.

What He has taught me about forgiveness and healing in this time, I wouldn't change for the world. I felt that time at Renewal was a huge turning point. I started to own mine and Teo's birth story. I started to see with fresh eyes the hand of the Lord in that delivery room, Jesus standing over us, guiding the surgeon's hands, surrounding us with angels that sang with every nurse and doctor in that room. I began to realise that that moment was a turning point, where God allowed the test to bring Martin and I to a deeper place of appreciation, of worship, of trusting and loving each other in Christ.

The blessing far outweighed the trial. I have nothing to complain about. Our daughter is alive. There are so many stories I know where babies don't make it, where mothers have to deal with the sorrow of not hearing their child cry.

Everyday, I had to make a choice to forgive, to heal and to lean into the abundant life Jesus talked about. Forgiving my body for "failing", my blood pressure for being too high. Forgiving that GP who told me it was my fault she was early because I was fat! True story. Forgiving all the professionals when I felt my aftercare was no way near what I needed when I didn't understand how my body should heal. Forgiving those who said my milk wasn't enough and that I needed to change strategy. Forgiving the health visitor who said to me, I needed to stop reading and doing my own research and just listen to her about Teo's development. The list goes on and on.

At each of those battle moments, the Lord was inviting me to a deeper place of letting go, dealing with pride and receiving a truth about me and my family. Those were battles for deep healing. Google, doctors, professionals, health providers only know so much. You know who knows your child better than you? God Himself. Do you know who is writing their story? God Himself. He knows the plans He has for them.

One of my concerns was Teodora's development. Because she was premature, I read every book I could find about how prematurity might affect a baby. The statistics and figures can be quite grim. The earlier your baby, the more likely they will have a delay to their motor development, a problem with one of their functions - breathing, digestion, sight. The list is scary. Once again, the enemy tried to use this to intimidate me and hinder my prayers.

Each baby is so unique, so different. Such a miraculous gift. There were nights, I cried out to God because at four months I hadn't seen her roll, by ten months she was only army crawling, she seemed to have no interest in wanting to stand up. I calculated everything based on her corrected age and still she didn't necessarily meet milestones when science said she would.

What underpins a mother's motives in sharing how quickly her baby does something? It's a narrative that she is a great mother because her child has achieved something ahead of the others.

Ouch! There is again. Pride. Once again, the invitation was there to let go of my expectations of motherhood. In many ways, the Lord has had to undo many years of a teacher's mindset. There is nothing wrong with being goal-oriented and setting targets, but when that becomes a defining feature of our identity, sooner or later it becomes an idol of success that God doesn't not tolerate. He didn't want me to be that way with Teodora.

I am learning the beauty of reading her for who she is and who God has made her to be. I am learning to embrace observing this little person unfold, grow and develop before my very eyes. It is like becoming a teacher all over again. Everything I knew about planning and preparing for children in a classroom is exactly that - for a classroom. Everything I am learning about being a parent is more a milestone for me in humility than it is about Teodora's own developmental milestones.

Fifteen months on, I needn't have worried so much. The joys of her emerging playfulness and cheeky smiles prove to me she is doing more than fine. Martin and I keep a book of funny things she does, in the hopes that one day we'll look back and remember her early days. We wrote down how many words our 15-month old now says. She may not have walked early, but she sure did start speaking early. I could sit and analyse how me and Martin taught that or brought that out of her.

The truth is, we didn't plan for that. We didn't sit and come up with a programme of getting our baby speaking early. I believe it's a combination of who God has made her to be and what comes naturally to us as parents to model. I'm learning to chill! Wow, first time mothers can really be anxious and full of second guesses. Does God give me a developmental milestone list of how my spiritual relationship should progress? Certainly not. It grows and is nurtured in relationships. I reflect what He has given to me.

From the very beginning, God has been showing me, Martin and Teo how to grow in our relationship as a family. The enemy of our souls has a plan to confuse, derail and lie to mothers, to steal their mandate as nurturers, stamping out their instincts to comfort and observe what their baby needs. The truth is that the Lord knows you are ready for children before you do. He knows what you can take, He knows your capacity for loving a child before you do. You are more than capable with Christ's help to be a blessing and example to your children.

Children are a blessing from the Lord. With this one child, I already feel so enriched and so fulfilled. My life is filled with a renewed vigour and purpose to live for God in a way that builds a legacy for our family. Who knows what He will do next? I know there is much to learn and much He wants to do through us.

This past year has given birth to a beautiful, talented and special little girl whose future is full of promise and God's delight. This year has birthed a mother who is learning everyday to humble herself before Almighty God and seek Him for the life of my children.

A prayer for you Mama

Lord Jesus,

I pray for the precious mama holding the pages of this book. I thank you for her life, for the woman she is and the joy she brings you! Thank you for the heart you have given her to raise her children, champion her family and love her husband. I ask that you would give her a fresh revelation of the story you have written in her about the mother she is and the gift she is to her family.

Where she feels she falls short, show her how awesome and how strong she truly is. If there are traumas and questions from the labour of her baby/ies, would you show her how you were there through all of it. Take away any fears or worries about how she raises her child/ren, show her that you are the Father who provides all she needs and that by your Holy Spirit you nurture, comfort and teach her how to follow you in her family.

When she feels tired and overwhelmed with juggling responsibility and spinning many plates, show her Jesus, how you understand, show her that even in the mundane you are weaving a rich worship and praise into her household. When she feels she can't give any more and she is drained from pouring out, show her that she cannot out-give what you give to her - your vast supply of love, grace, patience, peace, hope and strength. Thank you Lord, that you do not give to us more than we can bear and that in every season, you are God with us! You are God through us!

I pray that in her family, the testimony of your salvation, healing and deliverance would give you great glory and that when her children are grown up, she will say, they knew the Lord and they did not depart from His ways. Bless her household, bless the work of her hands, give her strategy and divine discernment to cover and nurture her children in prayer, godly wisdom and grace. I pray that when she looks back over the years of raising young children, she will see how you marked the days with your presence, how you richly provided, how you victoriously came through for them in every twist and turn of life. I pray that her testimony will be how faithful you are and how faithful you have been to her and her children.

Fill this woman with a fresh wind from the Holy Spirit, to run the race well and to press on to the upward call of Christ through raising her family.

In your precious name Jesus, Amen!

***With special thanks and unending gratitude to:**

All the doctors, nurses, midwives and staff at the NICU, HDU and Labour Ward, Newham General Hospital

Our church family who prayed and covered us in the Spirit especially River Church, The Revival Church and Commonwealth Church

Afia, Dorothy, Mark and Martin for being my sounding board, proof readers and design eyes

To my sisters in Christ who prayed for me as I wrote this book and encouraged me to write the words Jesus put on my heart - you know who you are.

www.ingramcontent.com/pod-product-compliance
Lightning Source LLC
Chambersburg PA
CBHW020243010526
44107CB00002B/78